Reverse your Age

Learn to Eat Healthy, Feel More Energy, Reverse Diseases, and Unveil the Best Version of Yourself

Your Practical Handbook To Look and Feel Younger

Written by Dr Maya Modi
**M.B.B.S, D.G.O, F.I.S.G.E.[U.K]
PGDMLS [PUNE], OZONE EXPERT**

REVIEWS

Dr. Rohit Bhatt
M.D, DCH, FAMS
[Renowned World Famous Gynecologist]
1, Shivani Society, Vasna Road
Chief.Dept.Ob.Gyn.BD, Amin Hospital
Baroda 390007

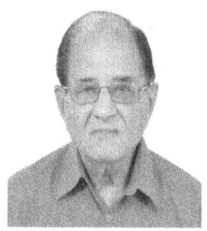

The whole universe desires to have a happy, healthy and peaceful life. Unfortunately, most people fail to follow the rules to lead a healthy life. World Health Organization [WHO] defines health as, "Health is state of complete physical, mental and social well being and NOT merely the absence of disease or infirmity"

Though longevity has increased in last few decades, modern lifestyles have given rise to many problems. These problems are due to consumption of fast food and other unhealthy diet, lack of adequate exercise, increasing stressful life and exposure to drug abuse, tobacco and alcohol. Modern life style has increased diseases like diabetes, high blood pressure, cancer, depression and many other diseases. This applies not only to elderly women but it affects man alike.

Dr. Maya has written the book mainly keeping the elderly women in mind. Therefore, I will comment only on issues related to women. There is increase in consumption of fast food which invites many diseases. Obesity has emerged as important life style issue. Depression is now on the increase in women sometimes leading to suicide. Lack of adequate exercise and stress increases health problems. In one small town in Japan, there are people who live for more than 100years in good health. The often quoted Japanese word IKIGAI means mental state in which individual feel at ease and remains active. Bhagwat Gita in chapter 6 gives sound description in to remain healthy. Lord Krishna tells Arjun that adequate sleep, not too much food or fast, remain active in purposeful activity is the key to good health.

Most women wish to know how to lead a healthy and peaceful life but they do not know where to get the relevant information and guide lines. Dr Maya is a doctor herself and has made intensive study of various types of foods which need to be consumed to remain healthy. She herself is not only preaching but has shown by example how to obtain bo`dy figure. The book gives very detailed information about various commonly consumed foods, their calorie values and usefulness.

I feel the information about meditation and various exercises have added value to the book.

However the detailed information about various food items serves great purpose.

This book may serve as a Bible / Gita for all women who wish to maintain good health at all times. It may also be useful to health care providers while advising their clients.

Rvbhatt

Dr Rohit Bhatt. 15/12/2020.

……….   ………

Dr. Pankaj Desai

He is an eminent obstetrician and gynecologist. A well know faculty of India and abroad. He is literary person and has written a book on post partum hemorrhage and is a best seller.

It was since 1971 that the obesity pandemic has gripped the world in its vice-like grip. If one compares the photos taken in the years before 1970 with those taken now, one would immediately notice many obese and overweight individuals in recent pictures. It is estimated that there are more over-nourished individuals than under-nourished on this planet. Not until recently, has the big secret behind the global pandemic of obesity tumbled out. It has been found that sugar in any form and heavily processed food together has contributed most to the weight boom. I was shocked to know that our popular colas which many of us drink so casually can have up to 44 spoons of sugar in a litre. When such a dire situation has unfolded, the wise always advice avoiding consuming foods about which you do not know what has gone into their making.

This automatically opens up the need for a book like the present one. The hard work and the scientific knowledge that has gone into the making of this book is its strongest USP. Very carefully written chapters loaded with necessary and guiding information about our foods and their components makes this book an information-storehouse for the reader.

I am sure that the readers 'misbeliefs' would be scientifically cleared as they will go through it. If you are concerned about your health, if what goes in your body in the form of food matters to you, if you do not want life-style diseases to catch you early – then this is an excellent book for you.

www.drpankajdesai.com

········· ·········

ACKNOWLEDGEMENTS

I Dedicate this Book to my
Mother and Son and Others
My Mother Padmaben Jayantilal Shah
My son Dr. Setu Bhagirath Modi [both my inspiration]
Saudamini Bhagat who helped me to write correctly,
My brother Harish Shah and Prayag Shah

And various women in their different phases of life to

Walk through life without a stick.

. My mom and son are the real accurate role models in showing that foods-are your pathway to health and my inspiration to write this book. Their teaching and values have played a significant role in striving me to be where I am today and become strong and healthy. Their full guidance and

support in my endeavor has filled me with joy and happiness. I express my deepest gratitude to them and I dedicate this book to them. Special thanks to Saudamini Bhagat teaching and correcting many phrases and sentences, without whose help I would have been lost. My brother Harish shah and Prayag Shah deserve a special mention. Harish has been with me consistently and Prayag has been my laptop help without whom I would not have hit the publication button. I am grateful to all those women who have motivated me on this journey and all those who gave me the strength. Too many women in their various phases of lives to walk though me without a stick. Those who all have given me the strength to dream high and fly high and achieve my goals. Their positivity and teachings have guided me and made me feel precious and significant.

This book's accomplishment would not have been possible without the guidance of mentor and friend, Som Bathla. I am grateful and thankful to him.

Dr. Maya Modi

drmaya53@yahoo.com

Do give your reviews which matters a lot.

CONTENTS

Reviews			2
Acknowledgements			7
Introduction			13

		Part 1	
Chapter 1		Why This Book	26
Chapter 2		Changes In Human / The Real Aims And Objective	37
Chapter 3		Essentials Of Life Water And Macronutrients	43
Chapter 4		Other Essentials Of The Body	67
	A]	Adaptogens - *To Increase Energy And Reduce Stress*	
	B]	Free Radicals Damaging Circle To Health	
	C]	Antioxidants - *Fountain Of Youth*	
Chapter 5		Trace Elements Of The Body	74
	A]	Copper - *The Dimer Of Health*	74
	B]	Magnesium - *The Cell And Muscle Vitalizer*	76
	C]	Zinc - *Adjuvant To Increase Blood*	79
	D]	Omega-3 Fatty Acid - *Oils Of Our Body*	82
	E]	L - Carnitine - *For Weight Watchers*	85
	F]	CoQ 10 Enzyme - *As An Adjuvant Therapy*	87
	G]	MSM - *Joint Lubricant And Wrinkle Reducer*	88
Chapter 6		Spices & Herbs	91
Chapter 7		Fruits - Their use in Diabetics	105
Chapter 8		Vegetables & Greens	116
Chapter 9		Nuts - Nuts Are Hard To Crack, Nut You Are Not!	132
Chapter 10		The Hunger Inhibitor - *Leptin & Grehlin:* Appetite Suppresser & Appetite	140

Increaser
Adiponectin- *Fat Burning Hormone & Regulates Glucose Levels*
CCK: Empties Your Stomach Quickly
PPY: Makes Stomach Full Easily
GLP: Increases Insulin Release

Part 2

Chapter 11		Foods For Different Parts Of The Body	149
	A]	Foods For Skin, Overall Health - *Keep The Skin Wrinkle Free*	150
	B]	Foods To Increase Collagen - *Keeps The Skin Tighter*	159
	C]	Foods To Reduce Inflammation - *Satvik Healing*	170
	D]	Foods For Eye - *A Better Sight*	175
	E]	Foods For Hair - *Strong Hair*	177
	F]	Foods For Gums And Teeth - *Healthy And Shiny*	179
	G]	Foods For Mouth Ulcers - *How To Avoid And Treat It*	181
Chapter 12		Don't let My Heart, My Diabetes, My Blood Pressure come into you	183
	A]	Diabetes	184
	B]	Hypertension / Blood Pressure	196
	C]	Heart Health - *Cardio Vascular Diseases*	198
	D]	Obesity - *Obesity Kills*	201
Chapter 13		Foods To Maintain Your Iron	205
Chapter 14		Don't Be Crappy With Muscle Cramps	211
Chapter 15		Foods for Fatigue - *Pep Up Your Energy*	215
Chapter 16		Foods for Nails - *The Showy Healthy Nails*	218
Chapter 17		Food For Under Eyes - *The Dark Circles*	222

Part 3

Chapter 18	Night Armor - *Sleep Better And Smarter*	226
Chapter 19	Supplements - *The Need Of The Hour*	233
Chapter 20	Happiness - *But Smart Happiness*	241
Chapter 21	Exercise - *Another Breather Of Life*	247
Chapter 22	Meditation - *Bring Peace And Calm To*	255

	Self	
Chapter 23	Ikigaii - *Learn The Japanese Way*	263
Chapter 24	Ozone - *The Oxygen Needed For The Body*	266
Chapter 25	Alcohol and Anti Aging Juices	268
Chapter 26	End of Story - *"Don't Eat This Box*	277
Bibliography		286
Connect To The Author		288

INTRODUCTION

Let Food Be Thy Medicine
And Medicine Thy Food

Hippocrates

Food Plates To Live/ Liven Your Life
Healthy Digestion, All Is Well When Gut Is Well.
Functional Foods To Ease Arthritis, Burn Fat, Decrease Appetite

Life's Teachers:

Life And Time Are The World's Best Teacher.
Life Teaches Us To Make Good Use Of Time
And Time Teaches Us The Value Of Life

Dr APJ Abdul Kalam

Since childhood we all have a teacher or a guru whom we look up to. We learn many things from them. Who would you think are your gurus or teachers? Like charity begins at home. Same way our teaching starts with our parents and the teachers. Life itself is the outstanding teacher of all; it has a way of teaching us things differently. School teachers and parents play a vital role in the holistic development of the child. Parents are the first mentor of the child and the teacher is the second mentor of the child. Both contribute immensely to developing and shaping their lives.

My best teachers are my mother Padmaben Jayantilal Shah and my son Dr. Setu Bhagirath Modi.

My mother Padmaben Jayantilal Shah is 87 years old. She still has the same grace, smile, body, and hardly any changes in weight. She moves about and does her daily routines easily.

She has had seven deliveries, and in spite of this she is in shape. She has a very small soft abdomen, with any fat in it. We all would be ashamed to see this ageless beauty.

She has regular meals. Her weight has constantly remained at 48kg. She always had breakfast, lunch, tea, and early dinner. She was and is a stickler of principles. If she weighs herself on the weighing scale and finds that her weight has increased by one kg, she would immediately stop sugars, ate much less for a few days, in order to balance the weight. She owns it and is still doing it. She would not wait for few more days. She believed in prompt action. She says in the end we only regret the chances we didn't take.

She eats only freshly cooked foods and no left over's. She chews her food well and teaches me the same thing. She keeps her interval of foods properly spaced. Her food plate is always nutritious and never indulged in overeating. She is not fond of fried foods, which is a good thing.

When my mother was young, I had just entered the medical college. Due to my teachings at M.B.B.S. Level, I was giving her calcium, Vit-D3, Vit-B complex, and multivitamin. This helped to maintain her health. She likes to work round the clock and advises not to sit after your meals. She would sleep only after an hour. I did her various pathological tests, especially blood sugar, thyroid profile, hemogram and cholesterol. They were done on regular basis. Due to her own self care in foods and medicines, and her walking habits, have helped her to stay fit and strong.

My son Dr. Setu Bhagirath Modi is a big inspiration to me. He has had a great weight loss of 25 kg and the best part is he has maintained it. He has achieved this over a period of two years. He realized that exercise is vital but even still more important is the regular small meals. He says Mom it is 80/20, meaning 80% is foods, and 20% is exercise.

It was really hard work for him. He works 9 to 10 hours a day. Yet he would always take time to exercise. If he is not able to exercise he would end up walking his pet Groot. He formed a daily habit of it. But afterwards everything was streamlined easily. He says life will only change when you become more committed to your dreams and goals.

He is very fond of food. Yet he is controlled his mind in not overeating the foods. He says you either control your mind, or your mind will control you. So similarly if the foods control your mind, it would be a death sentence of your life. There enters all the illnesses crouching your heart to drowning your mind body and soul. He tries new foods every day. He is fond of chicken, sea food and prawns with lots of salad and its ingredients. He opts out for small meals with healthy toppings and literally two tea spoons full of oil a day.

He tells me mom, input and output is important, only then the fat can burn otherwise it is accumulated on the body in odd areas and makes you look ugly. He says anyone can work out for an hour, but to control what goes on your plate the other 23 hours is the game changer. That's where the hard work is!

Setu says that what you burn can be expressed as a number of calories. He always insists on consuming adequate amount of water, without which there is trouble in digestion and health. His health is good and he gets compliments from people very often. He says cook your own meals and use ingredients to make it tasty. Never starve yourself. Incur vegetables, salads and fruits in your daily habits.

Remember, My son says - Being healthy is not about eating less. It's about eating enough of the right things. *That is - Only You Can Do It.* Old is gold means that the old things are very important and valuable. We should not think old is a waste. The foundation of all new things in the present world was laid in the olden days and what we are getting at present is all updated. It is the old inventions which form the base of the new ones. So we need to value the old things much as these are the basics of learning new things.

Old is a combination of "Old" and "God"

Once upon a time a giant ships engine failed. The ship's owner tried one expert after another, but none of them could figure out how to fix the engine. Then they brought in an old man who had been fixing ships since he was young. He was able to solve the problem by a combination of experience and ingenuity. Similarly one has to reinvent in oneself.

Health Journey Begins

Why should you embark on this journey? Many questions are hovering in your mind. You may know, you may not know the methods, and other people and despite knowing everything ignores the signs.. Health begins with your mind body and soul. If your body is not in proper condition, then how is your mind going to work. So now is the time to walk through life working your way to health?

Health and Ageing

HEALTHY CITIZENS ARE THE GREATEST ASSET A COUNTRY CAN HAVE

Winston Churchill

Ageing and health has become a global concern by World Health Organization [WHO]. The poor nutrition and diseases are a concern to health, and a cause of great concern. Causes of ageing include, but are not limited to oxidative stress, glycation, telomere shortening, side reaction, mutations, aggregation of proteins, etc. in other words, it is the progressive damage to these structures and functions that we perceive and characterize as ageing.

Age is just a Number

Age is just a number. It is all in the mind. The intelligent mind teleomeres the signals into thoughts, as to what you are thinking?

Are you wondering about your aging and its effect on your body? In fact, as the Author calls it - think out of the box, as to how you can be free of diseases. Walk your way till you embrace death and combating and defeating the disasters in your life.

An attractive aging model is based on the interaction between the processes of generation of damage or, as the author calls it, deficits accumulation, and the decrease over time in damage control and recovery. It is the round and round occurrence of a "vicious circle".

Breaking the Circle of Damage to Health

Aging is not fatal and usually they do not die due to age but mostly diseases which are largely preventable. The concept of aging is a mistake. Aging is a routine procedure, but we embrace the wrong things in our lives. We are entrapped by the different disease which encircles us like a storm and we do not know how to get out of it. Aging is very little genetic. Suppose the life span of our parents is 90 years then we can add a few years to our lives only.

If you start early, you can reverse aging. Yes Aging is Reversible.

If you remove toxins from your body, remove stress, meditate, exercise you can see miracles. But the most adjuvant therapy is foods. You have to increase the antioxidants in your diet, which can actually reverse the biological markers of aging. Your hormonal levels will reverse and become normal. Your eye sight shows remarkable improvement and blood pressure reverts to normal. I have mentioned all the reasons in aims and objectives. So start by learning to have less stress, change your foods habits and remove toxins from your environment. This will give quality and quantity to your life. The scientific wisdom says [Dr. Dipak Chopra] Our biological potential is 130 years, which means till you are 70years you don't begin middle age. This is the best time of your youth. Rock it everyone, to these benefits.

Abstract Aging impairs senses and body functions causing diet insufficiencies and change in nutritional needs. The present needs of independent older adults suggests that health research and care should form reductionist disease management to integral and personal treatment plans, including nutritional, lifestyle and psychological coaching approaches. They should incorporate education of macro and micro nutrient needs to the elderly. One should incorporate nutritional plans early in the life of a person to postpone the fatalities and break the circle of damage to health.

Follow our Ancestors
Our ancestors always applied to food plates, less known in those days. They had the habit of eating home cooked food.
Home cooked food, made from fresh foods, and not saw the light of fried foods or sweets. The sweets and fried were special meals awaited on all festivals.

How many of us know the food recipes or even the ingredients that our grandmothers knew? They and their mother-in-laws, had to whip up meals for large joint families thrice a day, and there were no refrigeration. So actually eating seasonal fruits and vegetables were not a fashion but a necessity both in terms of what was available and also the cost of it. And this dependence on foods also kept alive their primordial connection with the elements, and made them mindful of our bodies' in the heat and cold, rain and dry weather.

We are taught through generations to follow our parents. But modernity has made us - the descendants of those intrepid ladies – dismissive of the world around. Technology and cold chains have made anything available anywhere at any time. And worst still, globalization has made us hanker for, and also prefer, vegetables and fruits not suited to our land, or possibly, us too.

As we look to organic for everything from food to clothing, it is also time we [re]turn to indigenous. We need to re-embrace the traditional bounty of our land, what was grown in the seasons and in turn what is uniquely suited to our physiognomies. We need to rediscover our grandmother's recipes for food and life itself.

Why Foods, Macro and Micro Nutrients

When a child is born, the mother feed the child with milk, and other vitamins and minerals for proper growth and development. The mother bestows all her care and love for her child and sees that he/she is fed well. Then why are we lagging behind. This is a global system. Why are we trying to be different?

Macronutrients are those nutrients that the body needs in large amounts. These provide the body with energy. Micronutrients are essential elements required in varying quantities throughout life to orchestrate a range of physiological functions to maintain health. Micronutrients support an array of critical biological functions including growth, immune function and eye function, as well as fetal development of the brain, the nervous system and the skeletal system. Micro nutrition deficiency is a form of malnutrition and a recognized health problem in many developing countries. Globally more than two million people live with vitamin and mineral deficiencies cited by Nutritional International. The world health organization added a multiple micronutrient powder of at least iron, zinc and Vit-A to its list of essential medicines in 2019.

There are certain hereditary diseases which to certain extent can be avoided and detected early.

Want to be Dependent or Independent: **In life dependency is going to take you down the road. Be dependent on one's own resources of efforts: Self reliance - if you won't help me, I'll manage without help. This has to be the spirit; it is within yourself only that can move you into action. So start putting your thinking box on and pledge for self help.**

On my own, I will just create, If it works, It works

If it doesn't, I'll create something else.

I don't have and limitations on

What I think I could do or be

This should be your motto.

Oprah Winfrey

Why Life is a Journey

One has to process through different phases of life childhood, adolescence, adulthood, the mid adulthood and seniors. One becomes a parent and grandparents. We all know that once our children grow up and get married, we are left alone: not in real sense. The younger generation is getting busy in their own lives. We are now free of our responsibilities and now have plenty of time to wile. This is the time for self realization and to invest in health.

Many speak as though they know everything, but as we age we become ignorant as a child. Many are unprepared for the road ahead. The spot light no longer shines on you. The journey might be with or without illness. Now the ball is in your court. Be prepared to eat healthy and walk without support, rather than hit the bed with illness. You will have to learn to live alone, to enjoy embracing solitude and being healthy. The road is rocky but never too late to start a new.

Let go off your attachments and prepare yourself mentally for the new phase of life. The way of nature and natural foods is the way of life, just flow. Any time of life is a good start. Just press the button.

So leave nothing for latter. The Moment Is Now.

Are Food Habits are easy to form?

First Forget Inspiration

> Habit is more dependable
> Habit will sustain you
> Whether you're inspired or not
>
> OCTAVIA BUTLER

Deep fruits give better results. It takes 21 days to make/or break a habit: Foods that are transforming and recipes out of your mother's kitchen are easy to adapt and incurred into your day to day practice, goes a long way in life. There is a popular method to build habits. It is called the 21/90 rule. The rule is simple. Commit to the food changes in your life to a goal of 21 straight days. After three weeks, continue for another ninety days. Thus the pursuit of goal will become a habit. Once you have established that habit, you continue nonstop and will have no problem to incur the habit lifelong. Just follow it and success will be at your feet. It is all in the mind so set a good mind set.

My father Jayantilal Shah taught me persistence and perseverance as the motto of life. Due to this habit I have crossed many hurdles in life.

Let's stop the no pain, no gain approach to eating: We need to stop this No Pain No Gain in food habits. We all go into the habit of cutting foods, alcohol, or stay on liquids. Then we think we need to maintain that weight. There is nothing like maintenance. Healthy eating is not like the Olympics, where you train and sacrifice for one pinnacle.

Life Changing Moment

If you have diabetes and your doctor puts you on medication to get your blood sugar under control, you will still need to stay on medications to keep them there.

The same goes for general health, but in this case, "your medication" is your lifestyle.

Let's face this, it all sucks. They make you fell miserable and in few weeks you gain weight.

The third "Secret" is pleasure. It is nothing like women laughing alone with foods / salad; it actually means enjoying your food.

If we are into it for a long time, we need to enjoy and have fun to help us sustain.

Enjoy the occasional cupcakes/dark chocolates too.

Just follow the 80/20 rule: yes, you should aim to be eating your vegetables, lean proteins, healthy grains and healthy fats 80% of the time, but allow that 20% sometimes to maintain balance.

PART 1

CHAPTER 1

Why This Book

The Journey Begins

THE FIRST WEALTH IS HEALTH
BY RALPH WALDO EMERSON

My schooling days at Sophia High School, Mount Abu

The story starts from my childhood days. One which was fun filled and was full of energy and enthusiasm. The habit of eating was fun but the expenditure in form of energy was good and amazing. One never realized these effects and was achieved very easily. Being a sports woman, playing basketball, volley ball, throw ball was fun and also what I ate was all utilized. It was always fun time with output of high basal metabolic rate. So there were no worries regarding foods and its effects.

Becoming a Doctor

As a youngster, I had many hopes and aspirations. One think was stuck like gum in my mind was that I wanted to become a doctor. My father also wished that I go into medicine for he wanted all of us to have a good degree. Unfortunately my father had studied up to 4th Grade due to his family circumstances. I at that time was offered a role in a movie, from none other than famous film star Rajkumar. I refused it, for my head was filled with dreams of becoming a doctor and the white coat fascinated me. I was also offered a modeling assignment, but that too, I rejected it. How could I dissatisfy and shatter the dreams of my father. Here I started realizing the effects of nutrition and output on the body. My figure was the envy of all and was compared with Aruna Irani the actress. But yet my mind was only set on becoming a doctor.

With determination and hard work and dedication I graduated to become a gynecologist. At this time there was no worry about food habits as we had to work unlimited hours. But as my journey as a practitioner started and came across women whom I treated them at different stages of their lives showed so much of structural physical and mental changes. That realization daunted on me and was trying to search for answers. Are these the same women? Why so much difference? I put on my thinking cap on and started analyzing as to what may be the cause. Thus the author's journey began, very early in life in search of health and fitness.

I now put my Authorpreneur Journey to test. As a gynecologist in my practice, I saw women in my OPD [Out-Patient Department] on regular basis. I started scrutinizing them and made a flow chart. The changes in them at 30 - 40 - 50 years of age seemed very unrealistic. I would even compare them to their friends and even actresses. I was fazed and dazed. Are these the same women that I had previously seen? They were deshaped, tyres popping out, diabetic and decreased interests. I never wanted to be one like them. So my research started, for the subject and its effects on humans always fascinated me.

So my interest in the subject of nutrition and health increased. My mind started ticking and went on to lateral thinking about it. My quest started by inquiring into their daily food habits, exercise, work, family time and interests. I noted that the amount of food intake was the same, as to what they ate, when they were young. Due to family work they had no time for themselves, and also a sedentary life style was adopted. Thus, I decided to go deep into the subject and my journey began on food and nutrition and its effect on health.

I was, and am, and was a fitness freak. I learnt aerobics online and from friends. Being a doctor, I was well versed with the joint and muscles movements of the body. Then, I learnt the role of nutrition from my friend Siri Nair. I learnt facts, that could change the body to energize, walk your way to health, to maintain weight, and obtain stunning looks at different stages of my life.

I started experimenting different foods for the different parts of the body, and was surprised at the results, I obtained. I started getting compliments for my face, my energy levels, body structure, etc. The best compliment came from an old friend whom I had met in 2009. Her words to me were - you are looking more young today [year 2020] then as to when I met you 11 years back. Today 4/12/2020 Dr. Rohit. V. Bhatt [world renowned gynecologist] gave me the biggest compliment of my life. He said Maya you have maintained your health and incurred good food habits. Dr. R. V. Bhatt is my guru and teacher and praise from him means a lot to me. Dr. Pankaj Desai has been very supportive and encouraging in this journey.

Along with my practice I started my fitness studio which I named it as *Setu's Fitness Studio and Oxygen Bar*. I well knew the benefits of oxygen, and so I had specially created an oxygen chamber which I named as –'*The Oxygen Bar*'. I took four batches of aerobics along with my practice. *They were Transforming Them From Inside To Outside.* Transforming growth can only happen from inside to outside. *Self awareness - self help - self improvement - self motivation - personal development - inside out.*

Support System is Necessary

My students and I shared and had a two way pathway of communication and support. I gave a diet plan to all of them. At end of every week, I would discuss about what foods they ate and also the portion of it too. I taught them strategies as to how one can sustain themselves in their journey. Each one was supportive and helpful to each other, to be better and better each day. At the end they all were very happy with their transformation.

Oxygen [O2] is an excellent therapy for any person and at any age.

My Setu's fitness studio had an oxygen room, which I called it *'The Oxygen Bar'*, It was a small room with dim lights, a comfortable chair and with soft pleasing music. The oxygen would just flow in the room and you just have to close your eyes enjoy and be relaxed. It was a regular habit of mine to sit in this oxygen bar weekly. The results of oxygen are amazing and tenfold. Oxygen is very useful for the body and in this covid-19 all are well versed with the word oxygen. The body is detoxified with oxygen and in the advent the toxins, are thrown out. Due to replacement with the oxygen molecule in the bodies cells it also assists in reducing your joint pains, inflammation, clearing your chest and nose, energizing you and giving more strength pre and post workout. It also peps up the body the whole day. It is known as hyperbaric oxygen therapy but I named it the "Oxygen Bar".

oxygen therapy, came into existence way back in 1662, when a British clergyman and physician named Nathaniel Henshaw used a system of organ bellows with uni-directional valves to change the atmospheric pressure in a sealed chamber called a domicilium.

In India, the hyperbaric oxygen therapy started in 2000, in Delhi at Apollo hospital in a private sector. I started my oxygen bar in 2006. It is extremely beneficial in all condition in improving health, diabetic foot, cancer, respiratory disease, etc., and the list is endless.

All my strengths are due to the good food habits, vitamins and the oxygen bar spa.

My love for dancing was stayed on with me since childhood. I have performed on Zee channel for the mummy's special dance called *Boogie Woogie*. The judge was Javed Jaffery, an actor and dancing diva. I was also, India's top fifty dancers in 2015 in Dance India Dance Super Moms. This does need a special mention because, if you want to dance one's nutrition and fitness levels have to be good. Both go hand in hand. This all has inspired me to pen down my experiences and to help and teach and reach many.

I am a member of Menopause Society of India. I was the founder president of club 35+. It is a club for non doctor fraternity with the Menopausal Society of Baroda. Here all aspects of health are taught along with different competitions, updating women's health. I have taken weekly sessions of health and fitness and lectures on bone and heart health.

There is a saying by Deuteronomy Rabbah

> IN VAIN YOU ACQUIRED KNOWLEDGE
> IF YOU HAVE NOT PARTED TO OTHERS

Life Is A Learning Phase

We all know our whole life we end up learning new things every day. So did I. In this journey of mine, many of my colleague's lent their helping hand to me. One of them was a dermato plastic surgeon, Dr. Umesh Shah, the other orthopedic surgeon, Dr. Shandelier and a nutritional therapist Siri Naiir. This book was evolved, because we all need change. One needs a fresh perceptive that is enjoyable, feasible and manageable in your over committed busy lifestyle.

Fit Body

A modern lifestyle has fuelled one to look good and be in shape. A fit body is the new status symbol. We all want to feel and look good. The looks give us confidence and feeling good helps to pump our ambitious nature. Most of us have the wrong information on fitness. We believe extensive workouts, low calorie foods, muscle bulging and shapely body is the parameters of good health. A fit body is one, where you can climb stairs, walk without a stick, do daily routines without feeling tired, and yet ready to spend your energy on other activities.

Power of Nutrition

We are made from food. It may sound clichéd, but it's true: food is life. Food and its components are the basic substrate of our structure and our metabolism. Without food there is no development, no growth, no warmth, no movement, no reproduction, and no cognition. We consume different foods with their potential effects on the body.

So understanding the power of nutrition and nutrients is tenfold. If correctly understood and implemented in a simple way, it has the power to decrease the incidence of heart disease, blood pressure, diabetes, Alzheimer's, memory loss, bone loss and better immune system. It would increase your work efficiency, and prevent birth defects, increase mind power, and better quality of life. The degenerative diseases even cannot be afforded anymore.

It is better to prevent the disease rather than, only treating it. We know prevention is better than cure. Optimal nutrition vitamins and minerals play a vital role in our life, and also help to avoid diseases. It offers a powerful defense against the onslaught of degenerative disease and not to forget the skeletal system which is the backbone of one's structural body.

It is essential to maximize our health in all respects. Optimized health with nutrients diet, exercise, meditation and positive outlook to improves the quality of life and make these ailments a thing of the past.

The aim here is to be equipped with the knowledge suitable for your health requirements. The kitchen cabinet essentials so you are not strained and thus consistent in following the guidelines. I am *not a Gyan Guru*, but it is based on my personal experiences and knowledge that I have attained.

My Slogan is: Fit at 40 - Strong at 50 - and Independent at 60.

Battle with Working Hours

Having worked 16 hours a day and still, I had reserve energy to do more. I worked, exercised, danced and ate portion cut healthy foods. But this does not mean, I have not struggled hard to overcome all hurdles. The feeling that nothing is there and other times felt everything is there. The lows and highs are a part of the game with weight gain, depression and stress. But then, I battled my way to a good regime of fitness which included good dense healthy foods, exercise and dance. For me dance was very rejuvenating and de-stressing. Dance is mind blowing and I am a freak for it.

This is an optimal nutritional guide for you, which are the most beneficial foods and intake for all parts of your body. Think global, eat local and farm fresh, adopt the old system of our ancestors.

Our Honorable Prime Minister Shree Narendra Modi has started fit India movement. He also is speaking the same language for health. The author says just take the few simple steps, to get you going and stay motivated, keep smiling, be energetic and live healthy.

SHARE WHATEVER YOU HAVE, INCLUDING KNOWLEDGE.
"GIVE - GIVE - GIVE"
"My Heart Will Swell With Joy If I Can, Reach And Teach Many."

So energize your mind, strengthen your body, and enlighten your soul with foods, vitamins and minerals.

Self care is the best option. A few changes are required, and I am sure you can easily achieve it. Oh? Think - "Can I"? "Of Course You Can!"

Everything is important in our body. But I am going to take up the foods for different parts of the body and digestion, the importance of it and how it can make you into smart, stunning and healthy women. People will stop by to give you the admiring look. It is not only the looks, but each and every body part will be healthy.

I admire Sophia Lauren, Her quote -

"THE MIRROR OF YOUR HEALTH IS YOUR SKIN,
IF YOU DRINK IT SHOWS ON YOUR FACE;
IF YOU EAT THE WRONG FOOD YOU HAVE PIMPLES.
IF YOU TAKE CARE OF YOUR FOOD AND LEAD A HEALTHY LIFE,
YOUR SKIN WILL LOOK BEAUTIFUL"

SHE MUCH RATHER EAT PASTA AND DRINK WINE, THAN BE SIZE 0 [ZERO].

CHAPTER 2

Changes in Human

The Real Aims and Objectives

TO KEEP THE BODY IN GOOD HEALTH IS A DUTY, OTHERWISE WE SHALL NOT BE ABLE TO KEEP OUR MIND STRONG AND CLEAR
BY BUDDHA

What changers can you expect both physical and mental. Let's start from the top of the body. Some are genetic and some are predisposed.

Types of Changes Expected with Age.

A] Overall decline in Body System function.

B] Variable decline in specific organs and systems.

C] Different presentation of diseases and symptoms.

1] Eyes
   a. The eye develops Cataracts, which are common. The others are glaucoma, refractive errors and macular degeneration. A diabetic can hurt his retina, lose his vision.
   b. There are crow's feet at the edge of the eyes. [Fine lines or wrinkles]. The eyes become dry due to less production of

tears. The eye lenses become cloudier and vision in dim light becomes harder.

c. There is also itching of the eyes, watering of the eyes, focusing at a point becomes less accurate, night vision not as acute, need for brighter light. Watering of the eyes occurs very easily.

2] Nose
One develops lots of allergies, breathing difficulties, cold and polyps.

3] Ears
There is hearing loss and more wax in ears. The ability to hear high pitched sounds is difficult. The sense of clarity of the words is diminished

4] Taste and Smell
There is some loss of taste and smell as you age. This happens due to unpalatable food, loneliness, dental problems or unwillingness to cook.

5] Pain and Touch
With age the skin becomes sensitive and thinning of it occurs. This is due to loss of collagen, loss of fat, loss of pigment. There are more tendencies to develop bruises, skin breaks more easily. The body's ability to maintain temperature is decreased.

There is development of wrinkles more on the face and hands.

6] Teeth
The teeth decay easily. There is loss of teeth; and they fracture easily. The gums thin down and chewing becomes a problem too.

7] Face
Wrinkles on face develop due to loss of collagen and fat. Discoloration of skin and it becomes thin and fragile too. The structural change of face is due to loss of tissue and fat. Thus bruising and attack to heat stroke of skin occurs more easily.

8] Hair
There is Loss of hair, thinning of hair, rough hair, baldness, brittle hair.

9] Nails
Nails become brittle, ridges on the nails, blackness of nails, spoon shaped nails, clubbing of nails, scaling of nails, thickened fingers and also include the toe nails.

10] Skin
Skin shows: wrinkles, dryness, allergy, loss of moisture, pigmentation, rough skin, thinning of skin, Rugosity of skin.
The skin's ability to form Vit-D is decreased, when it is exposed to sunlight, thus the risk of Vit-D deficiency increases.

11] Breast
Breasts are first to show signs of aging. There is deshaping of the breast with change in contour and shape. Sagging of the breast occurs to the extent that it reaches your waistline.

12] Lungs
The lungs are at increased risk of infection. The trachea and central airway increases in size, there is decreased lung weight, and chest wall thickens, and increased risk of respiratory failure. Along with it there is loss of elastic recoil

in the lungs with decreased maximum expiratory flow.

13] Heart
The heart wall is known to thicken and maximal oxygen consumption is decreased. There is increase in heart rate and the systolic blood pressure increase at rest.
the blood vessels loses its elasticity and fatty deposits build in the arterial wall. This causes increase in blood pressure with [atherosclerosis] hardening of the arteries.

14] Gastro Intestinal System
There is narrowing of the esophagus and it contracts less forcefully as its musculature is affected. This leads to difficulty in swallowing. Hence there is inability to eat hard foods, and have to opt out for semisolid or less semi solid foods.
The intestinal motility is affected. This leads to digestive disturbances, constipation, infections, gaseous distension, gas, pain in stomach, and decrease of gastric secretions. Hence nutritional absorption decreases leading to fatigue, weakness.

15] Bones
First and foremost one will notice loss of height in inches, due to compression of the spine. There is stooping of posture, osteoporosis, osteoarthritis, arthritis, fractures, ligament tear. There is sarcopenia, which is loss of muscle mass and decline in muscle strength. This inevitably leads to fractures, fragility, reduction in quality of life and independence and osteopenia. Right type of diet and exercise will help.

16] Kidneys and Urinary Tract

The kidneys become smaller as you age. So the kidneys become less efficient in removing waste from the blood stream which leads to chronic diseases, diabetes and hypertension. There is more chances of developing infections, narrowing of urethra, difficulty in urination. The renal blood flow also declines.

17] Hormonal Changes

The deficiency of estrogen will cause fragile bones, atrophic vagina, and dryness of vagina, itching of vagina, ovulation and periods stop. Thus in menopause, mood swings, depression and irritability, weight gain, increased heart rate, fatigue, muscle weakness, irregular periods, hot flashes, breast tenderness, libido, insomnia, skin problems.

In males the size and firmness of the testes decreases and fibrosis may affect the penis, since erection is purely a vascular phenomenon. There is frequent and continuous urination which is a major problem due to loss of muscle tone.

In females due to hormonal imbalance there is frequent urinary infection.

18] Brain and Nervous System

The diseases are many. They are Alzheimer's disease, Parkinson's disease, neurogenerative disease, decline in memory, decline in co-ordination, reflexes are slow, slow movements, slow thinking, changes in sleep cycle [takes longer time to sleep] hours of sleep are decreased, sense of smell decreases and forgetfulness.

19] Weight

There is gradual increase in weight and in later years there is more of muscle loss. One shall become apple shaped.

20] Immune System

Here cancers are more common and vaccines tend to be less protective.

Summary

In many cases the decline that occurs with aging may be due to sedentary lifestyle, behavior changes, poor diet and environment. All this can be easily modified.

Taking steps to counter balance the effects of aging can help maintain a young spirit and independent life for which the first step is nutrition.

No person in their senses would like to harm oneself and end up in diseases.

You can always prevent the illness from to catching up with you.

Now is the time to say:

I SHALL - I WILL - I CAN

CHAPTER 3

Essentials of Life

Water and Macronutrients

Water

The water is the defining characteristic of health for your body. Don't ignore, drink plenty of water, and or fluids.

Alert for You

Everyone start or get into the habit of drinking water and fluids. Dehydrated cells work less efficiently. The cells that make up the heart, brain, lungs, liver and other organs of our body are unable to perform if they are not hydrated well. Dehydrated brain cells will cause fatigue. The skin will become dry and flaky. The recovery time from illness is delayed. Your overall ability to perform is decreased. So begin to understand the importance of water and hydrating nutrients. Water, milk, tea, juices, coconut water, soups, water rich fruits, water melon, musk melon, pineapple, peaches, Oranges and tangerine are some of the liquids to take to balance water deficiency. A combination of cell repairing nutrients such as essential fatty acids [EFA] and pomegranate extract. This water treatment has wonders effects on the skin's wrinkles.

Drinking satisfied my needs of water, but I needed to drink often and I am not diabetic. This was because my body was not utilizing the water. So to rehydrate my body I started having more nuts, eggs, soy and fish. Even if these were less I would take lecithin and EFA supplement every morning. Within weeks I was like a power house and working and cycling and having family time.

Don't ignore: One must drink plenty of water, and or fluids. The problems begin at around 50years of age. We have just over 50% of the water in the body and people over 50 have a *lower water reserve,* which is actually a part of ageing process. This occurs because the internal organs start responding differently. So to conclude people at 50 and above get dehydrated easily. It is not only they have smaller water supply, but they also do not feel the lack of water in the body. Although people at and above 50years look healthy, but their performance of reactions and chemical functions can damage the entire body.

Facts about Water

Drink water during the whole day - at least six to eight ounces of water per day. The athletes need more amount of water. Drinking sodas and coffee is not included here as these drinks makes you pee too much and acts like a diuretic.

Highly sweetened drinks are also not good as they are not easily absorbed by the body like water.

A diet high in fiber would require extra water intake.

The increasing age hazard is that, one ends up with less intake of water and illness knocks at your door. So everyone must pay attention to it and drink more water.

Drinking more water is good and will not bloat you up. Do not gulp water, but enjoy it. Salt and sodium rich foods, hormone imbalance and poor cardiac function are few causes of water retention.

Athletes should be cautioned that eating fiber foods like cereals, whole grain, and an apple before a workout will actually drain their water into the gut. Lack of water will significantly decrease your work performance.

Tap water contains a lot of chlorine which is harmful to our health. The other harmful elements are lead nitrates, radon and other toxic elements. This makes you more prone to heart disease, cancer, etc.

Summary: So all of you drink water throughout the day, and do not wait till you are thirsty. The habit of drinking water 2 hours after meals is healthy and your stomach does not get bloated.

Remember water is very important. "In one drop of water are found all the secrets of all the oceans and you"

Macronutrients

DREW CARREY SAYS:
"EATING CRAPPY FOOD IS NOT A REWARD - IT'S A PUNISHMENT."

Avoid these Foods as Food Matters

Spicy foods	Fatty foods	Juices	Alcohol	Carbonated drinks
Fast food	Baked goods	High calorie foods	High sugar foods	Preservative foods

Increase your salad, soup, grains, fruits, and cut to half the quantity of what you eat.

Other Essentials of the Body

Health is the New Currency

Macronutrients

Useful chemical substances derived from the food are called nutrients. Nutrients include fats, carbohydrates, proteins, water, vitamins and minerals.

10% fats, 25% proteins, 25% cellulose, 40% fruits and vegetables.

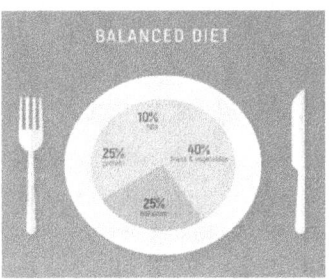

There are three main parts of the foods that the body requires.
They are fats carbohydrates and proteins.

TODD ENGLISH SAYS:
I USE A LOT OF SPICES, FRESH VEGGIES AND FRUIT, EXTRA VIRGIN OLIVE OIL, NUTS, AVOCADO, SOYBEANS AND ORGANIC INGREDIENTS AS OFTEN AS POSSIBLE.
WE NEED FAT IN OUR DIETS AND USING HEALTHIER FATS IS THE KEY.

Fats

Say no to theses foods

| Fried foods, deep fried | French fries | Doughnuts | Margarine | Burger |

foods				
Cakes, pastries	Processed snack foods	Crackers	Microwave popcorn	Foods with sugar
Margarine	Palm oil	Say no to these	Hydrogenated oils	French fries

There are of two types. These are saturated and unsaturated fats.

Bad Fats / Saturated Fats: Avoid These

Fats are Essential

The name fats itself triggers our mind, and thoughts as to, should I be eating it or avoiding it. Yes definitely, you need fats. But the kind and quality of the fat is more important.

Non-essential fatty acid is also known as body fat. This fat stores excess energy which can be used as fuel during starvation. Non essential body fat also protects and insulates the body.

Heart Healthy Fats

One type of polyunsaturated fat is Omega-3 fatty acids which have been found to have many positive effects. Polyunsaturated fats and monounsaturated fats will lower LDL ("bad") cholesterol when used in place of saturated fat. These unsaturated fats also help increasing sexual response, by raising the dopamine levels in the brain that triggers arousal.

Foods rich in these "good" unsaturated fats are listed below: Omega-3 Fatty Acids, alpha linoleic acid (types of Polyunsaturated Fat) *recommended by American Heart Institute

Fatty Fish 3oz/Week Should Be Taken	Salmon fish, Cod oil	Mackerel herring @ Tuna	Soy products
Sardines	Nuts, Seeds	Flax Seeds	Chia Seeds
Walnuts	Flaxseed Oil	Canola Oil	Brussel Sprouts

Polyunsaturated Fats (called Omega-6 Fatty Acids)

Unhealthy Omega-6 and Say Strictly No To Margarine

Palm Oil	Sunflower @ saffola oil	Cotton Seed Oil Soybean oil	Corn Oil

Healthy Omega-6 Foods

Peanut oil	Peanut Butter	Butter, Ghee	Olive Oil
Hemp Seeds	Sunflower Seeds	Eggs, meat poultry	Walnuts,
Walnuts	Almonds, Almond Oil	Tofu	Avocado

Vegetable Oils

Many of the oils are commercially refined, robbing them of their valuable nutrients. The Vit-E, lecithin is removed and stored in a glass bottle. Hence these oils have less nutritional value and are unhealthy for humans.

Hydrogenated Oils

They are extremely bad for health. In process of hydrogenation some of the healthy unsaturated fats are converted to Trans fatty acids. These Trans fatty acids are present in a wide variety of foods like bread, cereals, readymade dough, pastries, cakes, etc. The Vit-A is lost from the oils in the process of hydrogenation.

Pesticides in Oils

Most of the plants are sprayed with pesticides. On buying any oil ensure it is from a plant and not sprayed with pesticides or any other harmful products. Note the result of these pesticides is, we are adding a lot of pesticides into our body.

Margarine

Margarine is one of the hydrogenated oils. The process creates trans-fats that have a great destructive nature at a wider angle. These fancy, new fatty acids embark on your body and invade your metabolism creating havoc. The hydrogenated oils do not allow the production of prostaglandins and thus affecting your health. Margarine was originally developed as an animal feed. It is margarine in the west and Vanaspati ghee in Asian countries.

Are saturated fats the problem? They are found in dairy and meat and were blamed for various heart ailments. But this fact is actually false. It is a threat; in fact it is the margarines, vegetable shortenings and hydrogenated oils, which are to be blamed.

Recent Concepts

The recent concept is that butter, ghee, dairy products, and meats do not raise cholesterol and their consumption is allowed as previously advocated. The saturated fats are not to be blamed. They are essential part of your metabolism. If we ate no saturated fatty acids our body would make them.

It is only in recent times, that one experiences the use of hydrogenated oil, corn oil in many of the foods. Butter and homemade ghee are many times much better than margarine. Start using them especially in winters.

Unhealthy Fats / Trans Fats / Say No

Fried Foods	Stick, crackers, sausages	Baked Goods	Margarine
Microwave Popcorn	Hydrogenated Vegetable Oils	Readymade Dough	Ready to Eat Chicken
Fried Foods	Processed Foods	Cakes, Pastries	Oil Which Are Refined

Saturated Fats To Eat With Care

Fatty Cuts of Beef, Pork, Lamb	Poultry Skin, high fat dairy products	Chicken Wings	Dark Meat
Cheese, butter	Whole milk, sour cream	2% Reduced Fat Milk	Cream, Cream Cheese
Coconut Oil	Tropical Oils	Ice Cream	Cocoa Butter
Palm Oil-Say No	Palm Kernel Oil	Lard	

Trans fatty acids (or "trans fats") Just Say No and Only No. They are mentioned along with Trans fats.

Cholesterol

What about Dietary Cholesterol?

The Foods Listed Below Are Relatively High In Dietary Cholesterol™

Egg yolk or whole eggs. Limit to 2/week	Shrimp and squid / calamari one serving / week	Organ meats –liver, brain, kidney	Ice cream
Meat, Poultry, Seafood's are allowed in large amounts 5 or 6 oz / day.			
Mayonnaise	Mutton, meat crab	Sweet breads	Vegetable oils
Kidney, lamb, lrd	Cream half teaspoon	Cheese	Butter

Newer Study of Cholesterol

JANE BORCHERS, PREVENTIVE CARDIOLOGY CLINIC.

"NOW CHOLESTEROL IS NO MORE HYPED AND IT DOES NOT COME AS A MEASURE OF THE HEART DISEASE"

Gamma-Linolenic Acid [GLA] is often effective in the treatment of inflammatory diseases like asthma, arthritis, allergies, dermatitis and eczema. It helps to reduce premenstrual symptoms, like breast pain, bloating, depression and irritation along with helping in the mobilization of the joints.

Phospholipids

Phospholipids are water soluble and so they are hydrophilic. The fatty acids are hydrophobic [dislike water]. They effectively protect the inside of the cell from the outside environment, while at the same time allowing the transport of fat and water through the membrane. Phospholipids are ideal emulsifiers that can keep oil and water mixed.

Lecithin

Lecithin is found in honey, mustard and egg yolk, and is a popular emulsifier. Food emulsifiers play an important role in making the appearance of food appetizing.

Lecithin's crucial role in the body is clear, because it is present in every cell throughout the body. The 28% of the brain matter is composed of lecithin and 66% of the fat in the liver is lecithin. There is no need to take any pill for it.

Sterols

Cholesterol is the best know sterol because of its role in heart diseases. Cholesterol is used in the body to make a number of important things, including Vit-D, glucocorticoids, progesterone, testosterone, and estrogens. Notably the sterols found in plants resemble cholesterol in structure. However plant sterols inhibit cholesterol absorption in the human body, which can contribute to lower cholesterol levels. Though cholesterol is preceded by its infamous reputation, it is clearly a vital substance in the body that poses a concern only when there is excess accumulation of it in the blood. Like lecithin the body can synthesize cholesterol.

Prostaglandins

The fatty acids are turned into prostaglandins at every moment of your life. By ingesting healthy essential fatty acid the good prostaglandins are produced. These hormones are created at the site of injury and help the process of healing. Once blood clots they are no longer needed and the injury begins to heal. Another prostaglandin will stimulate the changes that allow the clots to dissipate and the blood vessels to relax.

In Women

Prostaglandins assist in regulating the reproductive system. They can start labor and control ovulation. They also have anti-inflammatory and immune-suppressing effects.

Important to Remember

Read the Labels of the Foods. - The labels on the food packets are very deceiving. Hence you should always read the contents for vegetable hydrogenated oils, sugars, corn oil.

Why to Avoid Fried Foods

A 100gm boiled potato = 87 kcal. While in the fried potatoes there is double the amount of calories.

Porous Foods

Food like sliced egg plant [Brinjal] is porous and when fried absorbs fat which amounts to 600 times more calories.

Surface Area

The potato wedges when fried absorb more oil than a whole potato.

Deep Frying

In deep frying of foods, fat replaces the water content of the food. At high temperature the water first evaporates and hot fat forms a crisp layer or crust on the food. Thus fried foods are difficult to digest.

Potato chips have added sugar, salt and hydrogenated oil. The carbohydrates here are a bigger issue than fats.

Packaged snacks and ready to eat should be avoided.

Desserts

Any dessert contain high amount of sugar.
The idea is to enjoy desserts once a week and in small portions.

Too much of proteins from meats are high in saturated fats.

Labeling on fast food packets and what is written is not always true. The bad oils are used which is harmful to health.

Energy drinks contains added sugar, plus ingredients that may potentially induce blood pressure or arrhythmia.

Added salt is there in many foods like pickles, chips, burgers, and chicken breasts that have been brained to stay juicy and moist. It is best to take less salt.

Which Oils are Good

Name of Oil	Temperature for the Oil	Uses
Peanut	320 Degrees	It can withstand high

oil	unrefined oil 450 degree refined oil	temperature. It can be used in daily cooking, stir fry, deep fry. Garlic, onions, and use of spices gives the oil more stability.
Flaxseed oil	225 degree temp for this oil. Not to heat but to pour and use it	It is used in stir fry, sautéing and for added flavor as a continent. It has omega 3 fatty acid. It is used as a salad dressing.
Canola oil	400 degrees	It is golden in color and pleasant tasting. It is low in fatty acids. It is used in all low heat recipes for baking, stir-fry, sautéing and roasting
Extra virgin olive oil	375 degrees	This oil is very beneficial. Good in taste. Can use in salads, dips and sauces.
Coconut oil	350 degrees unrefined oil 450 degrees refined oil	The refined oil is used in roasting and sautéing. The unrefined oil is used in baking and sautéing. This oil is very god for health. The edible coconut oil when take three times a day helps prevent Alzheimer's disease
Avocado cooking oil	Can be used at high temperature	It is used in baking, grilling. Add in a salad, as a smoothie.

As I have mentioned, the use of unrefined oil is better and made from ground nut oil, coconut oil. The use of ghee is most useful and helpful.

One should use ghee as and when necessary. Ghee is not harmful and it does not raise cholesterol. It provides essential oils to your body.

Summary

How much fat? You should get no more than 25% of your daily calories from fats, which should consist of non-saturated or polyunsaturated fats.

Weight Gain

Gaining weight from polyunsaturated fat appears to cause more gain in muscle mass than consuming a similar amount of saturated fat. A research from Uppsala University shows that saturated fat, builds more fat and less muscle mass.

Reverse for polyunsaturated fats. It builds more muscle mass and less fats in the body. The total fat intake should be less than 30% of total energy. This helps to prevent unhealthy weight gain in the adult population. The risk of developing diabetes and cardiac disease is lowered as well.

One should reduce saturated fats to less than 10% of total energy intake; and also reduce *trans*-fats to less than 1% of total energy intake.

How to reduce fat intake?

Fat intake, especially saturated fat and industrially-produced *trans*-fat intake, can be reduced by steaming or boiling instead of frying when cooking.

Use oils rich in polyunsaturated fats, such as soybean, groundnut oil, coconut oil, canola (rapeseed), safflower and sunflower oils. Homemade butter and ghee should be taken. One should avoid the foods as mentioned above.

My preference: I always opt out for less oil and boiled foods with herbs. I prefer taking ghee rather than other oils. Limitation is my key. I have gone off all fried foods and readymade foods. I just prefer home cooked foods.

Carbohydrates

Carbohydrates are our source of energy for immediate requirement.

ROBERT ATKINS SAYS:

A CONTROLLED CARBOHYDRATE LIFE STYLE REALLY PREVENTS RISK FACTOR FOR HEART DISEASE.

What Are Carbohydrates?

Carbohydrates are one of the three primary macronutrients that provide energy, along with fats and proteins. Carbohydrates are often classified as either simple (monosaccharide's and disaccharides) or complex (polysaccharides or oligosaccharides). Generally, complex carbohydrates have greater nutritional benefit than simple carbohydrates. The simple carbohydrates are sometimes referred to as Empty Carbs. Added sugars, a common form of simple carbohydrates, have little nutritional value and are not necessary for survival. While the body does require some carbohydrates (which are broken down into sugar), it is not necessary to consume sugary foods to meet this need.

How many carbs should I consume? The amount of carbohydrate intake varies depending on a number of factors. The *Institute Of Medicine recommends that a minimum of 130 grams of carbohydrates be consumed daily for adults. Other* sources recommend that carbohydrates should comprise 40-75% of daily caloric intake.

When carbohydrates are consumed in excess they are then stored as glycogen and are converted to fats. This acts as stored energy. In some cases when there is insufficient intake of carbohydrates and fats which are normally used as energy are not available. Then the body will start breaking down proteins instead, which can be very problematic. Proteins perform many essential functions in the body including serving as the building blocks for tissues and organs, driving many chemical reactions throughout the body, facilitating communication throughout the body, transporting molecules, and many more.

Good carbohydrates:

All Vegetables	Whole Fruits, pineapple	Apple, guava Banana	Strawberries, Papaya
Lentils	Kidney Beans	Peas	Pulses, Grains
Chia seeds	Macadamia Nuts	Peanuts, almonds	Hazel Nuts, walnuts
Watermelon, blueberries	Pumpkin Seeds	Quinoa, brown rice	Oats
Buckwheat	Sweet Potato	Oranges	Banana
Beetroot, carrots	Beans	Potatoes, tomatoes	Root Vegetables
Radishes Spinach	Sugar, Snap Peas	Turnips	Water Cress
Asparagus, lettuce	Fennel, herbs and spices	Garlic, onions	Brussel Sprouts
Broccoli	Grapefruit	Cucumbers	Cabbage
Peppers	Jicama	Clementine	Cauliflower
White Mushrooms	Kale, chare, celery	Broth of chicken, beef	Vegetable broth
Zucchini	Coffee	Tea	Water

Bad Carbs

Pasta, cereals, bread	Juices, soda	Canned fruits	Ready to eat yogurt

Cakes with frosting	White flour	Sugary drinks	Cookies
Pastries, pretzels	Fried foods	Chips	Pancakes with syrup
Cereal bar and candies	Ice creams	Milkshakes	White rice to eat in limited quantity.

Summary

How many carbohydrates a person consumes really depends on many personal factors. There are situations in which a low carbohydrate diet can be beneficial, even life-changing, for one person, but having a lower carbohydrate diet will not necessarily have health benefits for someone in a different situation.

The Dietary Guidelines for Americans recommends that *carbohydrates make up 45 to 65 percent of your total daily calories*. So, if you get 2,000 calories a day, between 900 and 1,300 calories should be from carbohydrates. That translates to *between 225 and 325 grams of carbohydrates*.

GARY TAUBES SAYS

THE POINT IS TO KEEP IN MIND IS THAT YOU DON'T LOSE FAT BECAUSE YOU CUT CALORIES; YOU LOSE FAT BECAUSE YOU CUT OUT THE FOOD THAT MAKES YOU FAT - CARBOHYDRATES.

How much carbohydrates you should be eating.
Who benefits from liberal carbohydrate consumption?
The recommended consumption of carbohydrates is 200 calories / day for a person who is physically active or lean or looking to build up body mass.

How to Manage the Carbohydrate Intake

Here one needs to take low starch veggies. (Different color vegetables).
Also take fruits - two helpings of fruits a day and along with it 3 to 4 cups of fibrous carbohydrates. Potatoes, wholegrain rice should be consumed in less quantity.
Who benefits from minimal carbohydrate consumption?
The allowance of minimal carbohydrate consumption is 100 grams per day.
This would be great if you are looking to get a jumpstart on your weight loss plan. So you can stick to eating lean proteins, vegetables, healthy fats, and minimal fruits.

What is a Good Start?

A good start is to aim for 1 gram of carbohydrate for pound ideal body weight. One can adjust up and down for weight loss but don't forget your intake of proteins and fats.

Note

Additional carbs are still important for muscle retention and fitness performance in endurance athletes and weightlifters. Carbohydrates taken pre and post workout can supply you with enough

energy and replenish your glycogen stores.
My preference: I have developed the habit of eating fruits. I eat seasonal fruits. Now I cannot do without eating fruits. I do not consume sugar. In fact I am using jaggery in place of sugar. I am happy using jaggery in tea. I avoid all sugary treats to myself. This I would take once a while. My meals do start with a salad daily with variant use of vegetables. I use carrots, cucumber, bell peppers, beet and sprouts in different forms. I love all vegetables and dals. I am off wheat and replaced millets. Millets are very good for health and diabetics. My saviors are spinach and eggs and sweet potatoes.

STRUCTURE YOUR BODY,
ENLIGHTEN YOUR FACE
THINK AND EAT HEALTHY
DR. MAYA MODI

Proteins

MARK E. HYMAN SAYS:
CALORIES FROM PROTEIN AFFECT YOUR BRAIN,
YOUR APPETITE CONTROL,
SO YOU ARE MOST SATIATED AND SATISFIED.

They are also called as First Place. The term protein is derived from a Greek word "Proteios" meaning "First Place". In 1839 a "Dutch Chemist "G. J. Mulder was first to describe protein.

Proteins in the body: They are the building blocks of our body.
They are the most abundant organic molecule of the living body system. They constitute about 50% of the cellular dry weight.

Proteins provide the long term energy when the carbohydrates and the lipid sources are not a available.

The proteins are of two types, 1] essential amino acids and 2] nonessential amino acids. The essential amino acids are obtained from food.

The non essential amino acids are made inside the body. The amount of proteins required for a person depends on weight, height and activity.

A person consuming 2000 calories will approximately require 100 to 110gms, provided a high intensity workout is done.
A person shall require approximately 56 gm of protein per day in divided doses, for an average sedentary man and 46gms for average sedentary women.

Protein makes up all living materials, like Alpha Keratin, 'ACTIN' and 'MYOSINE', haem protein. They are cellular construction worker, cellular messenger and helps maintain proper fluid balance.

Protein builds and repairs tissues, transports nutrition and provides other essential functions.

Utilization of Protein

There is a misconception that proteins are not good and they do not put on weight when eaten correctly.

Two Types of Proteins

The lean proteins are from non vegetarian foods. The non lean proteins come from vegetarian foods.

Vegetarian Sources

Chia Seeds	Hemp Seeds	Milk Soy Products	Rice and Beans, whole grains, lentils	Hummus, Pita Bread
Cottage cheese	Cashews, almonds	Chick Peas	Spinach	Peas, Beans
Amaranthe Natural Gluten Free Seed	Ezekiel Bread, it Contains 18 Essential Amino Acids	Peanut Butter Sandwich	Sundried Tomatoes	Buck Wheat, Quinoa
Spiraling	Grains	Nuts	Eggs	Pumpkin Seeds
Chana	Mooing Dals	Sprouts	Fenugreek Sprouts	Protein Powder

Non-Vegetarian Sources of Protein

| Chicken | Meat | Oyster | Lobster | Liver |

Turkey	Pork, beef	White Fish, tuna	Mutton korma	Salmon
Keema Dishes	Pamesan Fish Fingers	Eggs	Shrimp	Prawns with Mango

As per ICMR: 1 kg body weight for 1 gm of protein is essential.

Protein is one of the three main classes of food. They are made of Amino acids, which function as cells "building blocks. Cells need protein to grow and to mend them. Protein is found in many foods, like meat, fish, poultry, eggs, legumes and dairy products.

My preference: My daily routine is tea with jaggery and almonds soaked overnight. I always take different dals daily, some mango pickle and sprouts. Tomatoes and peanuts are a daily affair in consuming them. I do eat chicken sometimes. Eating eggs is a must for me, due to which my nails, hair and skin have improved.

Almonds and groundnuts I count and eat 7-10 daily.

Chapter 4
The other essentials of the body

A] Adaptogens

We use adaptogens to protect the body from stress and increased levels of cortisol.
They increase energy and reduce stress.
They are perfect examples of food as medicine.

Uses of Adaptogens

Tiredness
They help to decrease fatigue and anxiety.
They reduce stress and depression.

Hormones
They help balance hormones

Sex
They increase the sex drive.
They increase immunity and are helpful in cancers.

Foods with Adaptogens

Tulsi / Basil. It Relieves Physical and Mental Stress	Cordyceps Mushrooms, Boosts Stamina	Rhodiola: Here Physical, Mental Fatigue Is Relived	Indian Ginseng: It Boosts Memory
Astraglousroot Combats Fatigue	Licorie or Mulethe Will Reduce Stress	Turmeric Boosts Brain Function, Reduces	All Guidelines Only From Your

		Depression	Doctor

Ashwagandh reduces stress and anxiety.

Summary: To balanced and protect your body form stress one should take Tulsi, ginger, mushrooms, Ashwagandha and turmeric.

B] Free Radicals

The oxygen in the body splits into single atoms with unpaired electrons. These enter the body and get attached to other scavengers available to them. Free radicals are highly reactive and unstable molecules that are produced in the body naturally as a byproduct of metabolism (oxidation), or by exposure to toxins in the environment such as tobacco smoke and ultraviolet light.
They are the damage circle to health.
Free radicals have a lifespan of only a fraction of a second, but during that time can damage DNA, sometimes resulting in the mutations that can lead to cancer. Antioxidants in the foods we eat can neutralize the unstable molecules, reducing the risk of damage.

Sources of free radicals: lack of sleep, anxiety, depression, pollution, ultra violet radiation from the sun and cigarette smoking.

Effects of Free Radicals

Ageing,	Depressed	Cataract,	Inflamm

skin damage	immune system	cancer	ation, Hormone imbalance
Heart Disease	Diabetes	Senile Dementia	Atherosclerosis
Accelerates Nerve Cell Injury	Cause Damage to Part Of Cells Such As Protein, DNA, Cell Membranes	Cancer	Damage to Growth, and Survival of the Cells is reduced

Uses of Free Radicals

The body produces free radicals naturally. Thus sufficient amount of nutrients are essential to free these radicals. They help fight viruses and bacteria.

Free radical formation is crucial to the process of oxidizing nutrients from our food into chemical energy.

Tackling of Free Radicals

Antioxidants Such As	Vit-A, Vit-C, Vit-E	Protect damage caused by free radicals	Lutein, Polyphenols Cranberries Loaded With Them
Avoid High Glycemic Meals	Avoid Over Eating	Avoid Foods with Sugar, Carbohydrat	Limit Processed Foods,

		es	Sausages, Bacon, Salami
Don't Reuse Cooking Oil, Fats	Limit Alcoholic Drinks	Eat Antioxidant Rich Foods	Foods with Beta - Carotene, Lycopene Lutein
Brussel Sprouts	Carrots, tomatoes	Collard Greens	Egg plant, lettuce
Fruits Apples	Cherries, mangoes	Cantaloupe, grapefruit	Lycopene, Phytonutrients
Broccoli, alpha sprouts	Papaya, kiwi	Red Grapes, cranberries	Raspberries, strawberries, blueberries
Nuts, Walnuts	Sweet Potato	Flavonoids Such As	Onion
Endives	Pears	Red Wine	Turnip Green
Parsley	Cherrie, Berries	Limit red meat	Legumes, soya beans
Cheese	Tofu	Miso	Milk
Antioxidant Foods	Prunes, figs	Plums	Pomegranate
Oranges	Turmeric	Raisins	Sweet Red Bell Peppers
Beet	Kale	Spinach	Dark Chocolate
Grape seed extract	No smoking	Rosemary	Take teak which contains phenol

Other ways to tackle Free Radicals

Exercise

It pumps in more oxygen and hence less free radicals. Anxiety and stress increase free radicals and more diseases. Thus one must learn to remain calm and cool.

Eat Enough Proteins
The amino acids are products of proteins. One of the amino acid is glutathione which helps eliminate free radicals.

Adequate Rest or Sleep
Good sleep help fight free radicals by production of melatonin.
Adequate water: the elderly and athletes need to drink adequate water which helps to reduce the free radicals.

Don't Over Eat
Over eating produces free radicals. So incorporate healthy foods. And avoid high glycemic index foods. Foods with preservatives and processed foods also should be not taken. Eat food rich in flavonoids such as, onions, egg plant, lettuce, turnip, greens plumes, legumes, cheese, and tofu.

Take Herbs and Spices
Have ginger, rosemary, turmeric, ginkgo, grape seed extract, and tea which contain polyphenols.

C] Antioxidants

They are the fountain of youth

Antioxidants are called the fountain of youth. Antioxidants are substances that can prevent or slow down damage to cells caused by free radicals, unstable molecules that the body produces as a reaction to environmental and other pressures. They are Free Radical Scavengers. They help reverse aging and better quality of life.

Foods with Antioxidants

Vit-C Most Powerful Antioxidant	Artichokes	Onion, garlic, leek are the richest source of antioxidants	Raspberries, mangoes, Goji berries, tomatoes
Vit-A Carrots, Spinach Bell Peppers	Citrus Fruits	Vit-E in Nuts, Whole Grains, Bread	Parsley, Herbs And Spices
Cabbage	Beans, legumes	Beet, kale	Herbal Tea, coffee
Copper In Sea Food, Nuts,	Cruciferous Vegetables,	Foods with Beta-carotene Pumpkin,	Anthocyanins Group of Flavonoids Found In

Lean Meat, Milk	Cauliflower, Broccoli,	Carrot, Spinach, Parsley, Mangoes, Apricots	Grapes, Blueberries, Pomegranate And egg Plant.
Pomegranate juice	Coconut Water, yogurt	Green Juice	Catechins Are Found In Red Wine, Tea
Honey	Apple	Banana	Olive Oil

Pomegranate

Pomegranate symbolizes life and fertility. It has the strongest age proofing capabilities. They have polyphenols which are potent antioxidant. Ellagic is the most potent essential polyphenols.

To Remember

Pomegranate juice which had antioxidant has three times its effect. It is a most effective supplement. If pomegranate is not available then use its supplement.

Most important antioxidants are Vit-C, Vit-E, beta-carotene, carotenoids, manganese, Vit-B2, Vit-A, magnesium, zinc, copper, selenium, CoQ 1 enzyme, glutamine and taurine. But these are to be taken in a balanced form.

Antioxidants are the body's bodyguard.

Chapter 5

Trace Elements of the Body

A] Copper

The dimer of health

Uses of Copper

It is an essential nutrient in the body, and along with ion in the blood along with iron, it enables the body to form red blood cells which contributes to iron absorption.

Collagen

It is important for the formation of collagen in the structures, thus reducing the effects of ageing.

Synthesis

It aids in phospholipids synthesis.

Cardiovascular health

Low copper levels have been linked to high cholesterol levels and high blood pressure.

PROF. CHANG SAYS:
 "COPPER IS LIKE A BRAKE OR DIMMER SWITCH, ONE FOR EACH NERVE CELL."

His team found that, if high amounts of copper enter a cell, this would appear to reduce neuron signaling. When copper levels in those cells fall, signaling resumes.

Immune Function

Low levels of copper would also cause low levels of white blood cell.

Thus adequate amount of copper helps in maintaining immune system.

Bones

It maintains healthy bones, blood vessels and nerves.

Oxidation

Copper is part of the enzyme needed for fatty acid oxidation.

Hair

It ensures healthy hair.

Metabolism

Copper is needed for proper function of the body and its metabolism.

Deficiency of Copper

Anemia	Poor wound healing	Elevated cholesterol level	Neurological problems
Weakness paleness	Low white blood cell count	Connective tissue problems	Rare diseases Menkes disease
	Osteoporosis, bone fractures	Poor immune function	

Foods with Copper

| Coco | Winged Beans | Cashews | Squid, organ |

Beans			meats
Saffola Oil	Brazil Nuts	Sunflower seeds	Shell Fish, oysters
Yeast	Wheat Bran Cereals	Whole Grain Cereals	Chocolate
Cocoa	Dried Fruits	Black Pepper	Most of the iron tablets contain copper

B] Magnesium / MG

The cell and muscle vitalizer

It is the fourth important mineral playing a role of 300 enzyme reactions in the body. It is the second most abundant intracellular action in the body, 65% is in the bones, 34% in the intracellular space and only 1% in the extra cellular space.

Uses of Magnesium Energy

Magnesium is required by the cell membrane adenosine triphoshatase, the enzyme which supplies the energy required for the sodium pump.

Boost exercise performance

During exercise more magnesium is needed. Thus more magnesium helps better exercise performance.

Fights Depression

Magnesium plays a role in brain function and mood elevation.

Type 2 Diabetes

It is important in glucose control and insulin metabolism. It reduces insulin resistance.

Lowers Blood Pressure

It is helpful in people having high blood pressure and helps lowering it.

Anti-inflammatory Benefits

Adequate levels of magnesium help reduce inflammation and ageing.

Nerve and Muscle function

It maintains and *prevents cramps in the muscle*. It assists the nerve function.
Magnesium is used for making protein, bone and DNA.
Magnesium improves PMS [premenstrual syndrome] symptoms: It reduces water retention, cramps, irritability and tiredness.

Immunity

It supports the immune system.

Calcium and Vit-D

It helps to regulate calcium and Vit-D levels, thus one gets healthy bones.

Migraine

It may help to prevent and relieve headaches and migraine.
It also helps clear the stomach, so fewer amounts of toxins are built up.

Deficiency of Magnesium

| Muscle | Weakness, | Risk of | Fracture Risks |

Cramps Or Spasm	diarrhea, asthma	Osteoporosis	
Tremors	Poor Coordination	Loss of Appetite, nausea	Mal absorption
Hungry Bone Syndrome In Diabetics	It Prevents Bone Growth in Younger People	Cognitive Disorders, dizziness	Poor Memory, Alzheimer'
Depression, insomnia, stress			Restlessness
Constipation	Body Odor	Headaches	Poor Work Performance
Pre Eclampsia, Eclampsia in Pregnancy	Hypertension	Heart Disease	Increased Infections

Foods with Magnesium

Grains	Dairy Products	Bananas	Chlorophyll Rich Vegetables
Best Is Spinach	Roasted Almonds, Blackberries	Cauliflower, cabbage	Guava, raspberries
Cashews	Pumpkin Seeds	Skin of Potato	Avocado
Soy Milk	Cantaloupe	Low Fat Yogurt	Lima Beans
Quinoa	Dark Chocolate swiss chard,	Mackrel, salmon	Collard, turnip greens
Kale, Sweet Corn	Green Peas, okra	Artichokes	Acorn Squash

Magnesium Requirement

31 to 50 years males = 420mg. 1 to 50 years females =320mg.
51 years and above males = 420mg. 51 years

Above females= 320 mg.

Important: **The American College of Obstetrics and Gynecology suggests that taking magnesium supplement could help reduce, bloating, mood symptoms, PMS [Pre Menstrual Syndrome] and breast tenderness.**

C] Zinc

An adjuvant to increase blood

It is an essential trace element. It is second most trace mineral in the human body. Zinc is primarily an intracellular element; its content is thus proportionate to the lean body mass.

Uses of Zinc

Nearly 200 enzymes are known to require zinc for their activity.

Cell Division

It is present in all the body tissues and is necessary for all cell division.

DNA Synthesis

Zinc also has direct stimulating effect on DNA synthesis and replication, lymphocyte transformation and cell-mediated immunity.

Antioxidant

It acts as an antioxidant, fighting the free radicals damage and delay process of ageing.

Proteins

The body needs zinc to make proteins and DNA.

Immune System

It helps the immune system to fight the bacteria and viruses.

Fertility

It is important for fertility and for the estrogen and progesterone production.

Male Sexual Competency

Zinc helps produce key sex hormones such as testosterone and prolactin. Zinc also enables the main component of prostatic fluid. There is evidence that zinc may impact male sexual competency.

Body Needs

The body needs zinc during pregnancy, infancy and childhood.

Deficiency of Zinc

It is more common than is generally perceived.

Getting Sick Very Often	Feeling Tired All the Time	Decreased Fertility in Females	Poor Concentration or lack of alertness
Hair Loss	Delayed Wound	Early Ageing,	Unexplained

	Healing	stunted growth	Weight Loss
Decreased Sense of Smell, Taste	Decreased Appetite	Diarrhea, mal absorption syndrome	Open Sores on the Skin
Old Age	Alcoholism	Clay Eating	Excess Perspiration
Iron Deficiency Anemia	High Cereal Diet	Impaired Performance In School Children	Erectile dysfunction

Foods with Zinc

Red Meat	Poultry	Grass Fed Beef	Lamb, Oysters
Mature Dried Beans	Crab, salmon, chicken	Cow Peas, chick peas	Black-Eyed Peas
Cheddar Cheese	Cooked Oat Meal	Corn Flakes	White Wheat Bread Whole Wheat Bread
Turkey, salmon	Wild rice	Wheat Germ	Pumpkin Seeds
Cashews	Mushrooms	Cocoa Powder	Baked Beans

Zinc Treatment

Tablet zinc sulphate=35-120 mg daily in divided doses.

It is best administered with fruit juice, rather than with a meal high in phytate.

Raising plasma zinc levels with zinc supplements may reduce the plasma copper level, producing anemia and low white blood cell count.

This is corrected with supplement of copper 1mg daily as copper sulphate.

D] Omega-3 Fatty Acids = Fish Oil

Oils of our body

Fish Oil can be classified in two groups:
1] Those which store fat in the muscle [fat fish, such as mackerel, herring and salmon].
2] Those like cod which store fat in the viscera [liver]. Thus eating cod will provide very little oil, but liver of cod would be rich in oil; its high Vit-D content, however, produces toxicity and so prevents excessive use.
The three main essential omega-3 fatty acids are alpha linolenic acids [ala], epicos pentaenoic acid [EPA], docosa hexaeonic acid [dha].

Uses of Omega 3 Fatty Acids

It promotes hair growth and prevents hair fall.
Omega 3 helps with anxiety, depression, and memory loss.

Vision

It helps to improve vision.

Brain

Omega can promote brain health during pregnancy and early life.

Moods

Omega helps fight depression and anxiety.

Metabolic Syndrome

Omega helps lower blood sugar, blood pressure and obesity.

Children

In children it helps to reduce symptoms of ADHD, a behavioral disorder in children, and aids to lower risk of asthma too.

Inflammation

Omega helps reduce inflammation in the body, thus reducing heart disease and cancer.

Mental Disorder

In schizophrenia and in bipolar disorders omega-3 is known to control mood swings. It is also effective in age related mental decline disorder like Alzheimer's.

Heart : there is slow development of plaques in the arteries, thus helps prevent heart attack. It helps in lowering triglycerides.

Fish oil supplements do not lower high plasma cholesterol levels in middle aged men with=out elevated triglycerides.

Fish oil is beneficial in
a] Rheumatoid Arthritis

b] Reynaud's Phenomena

Fish oil supplements do not lower high plasma cholesterol levels in middle aged men with=out elevated triglycerides.

Fish oil is beneficial in
a] Rheumatoid Arthritis
b] Reynaud's Phenomena.

Important

High doses of fish oil are known to prevent platelet aggregation and produce bleeding.

Vit-A and D toxicity can occur due to fish oil consumption.

Increasing fish intake from 1-2 servings per week to 5-6 servings per week does not substantially

reduce the risk of CHD [Cardiac Heart Disease] among men who are initially free of cardiovascular disease. There are no signs and symptoms.

Foods with Omega -3 Fatty Acid

Milk	Walnuts	Chia Seeds	Flax Seeds
Soya Bean Oil, flaxseed oil	Canola Oil	Salmon, Herring Mackrel,	Caviar Consists Of Fish Eggs
Eggs 2eggs/Day	Cod Liver Oil	Oysters	Anchovies
Soy Beans	Meats	Dairy Products	Spinach
Sword Fish, Sardines	Tuna, Blue Fish. shrimp	Brussel Sprouts	Flounder, haddock

Dha / EPA Found In Wild Alaskan Salmon [Best], Cold Water Fatty Fish, Mackrel And Tuna

E] L-Carnitine3

For weight watchers

It is a naturally occurring amino-acid which is used extensively in weight loss.

It is a nutrient and a dietary supplement.

Our body can produce L-Carnitine out of the amino acids, Lysine and methionine.

For the body to produce L-Carnitine, one needs sufficient amount of Vit-C.

The body can convert L-Carnitine to other amino acids called Acetyl-L Carnitine and propiony-L Carnitine.

Uses of L-Carnitine

It has a good limited use for weight watchers.

Energy

It plays a crucial role in producing energy, by transporting fatty acids into the mitochondria cells.

Age Related

It helps age related mental decline and improves learning markers.

Brain

Helps the brain function better and improves decline of memory.

Heart

A potential to reduce blood pressure and inflammatory process associated with coronary heart disease.

Sports

It has good effects on sports performance. The recovery period after exercise is reduced.

Oxygen

It may increase the oxygen supply to muscle. Thus can enable increase muscle mass and reduce fat.

Blood

It may increase the production of red blood cells.

Deficiency of L-Carnitine

In Vegetarians	Frequent Dieters Low plasma carnitine levels	Medication for Seizures, irritability	On Dialysis
Tiredness, Hypoglycemia	Accumulation of Fat In Liver Muscles, Heart	Weak Muscles In Hip, Shoulders, arms, Leg, Neck, Jaw Muscles	Progressive Cardiomyopathy or Heart Muscle Disease

Foods with L-Carnitine

Beef. Beef heart	Chicken, meat	Pork	Milk
Whole Wheat Bread	Milk	Poultry	Fish

Important

Dairy products contain carnitine primarily in the whey fraction.

Requirement of Carnitine

150-500 micromol/ day
Carnitine needs a sufficient amount of Vit-C to be produced in the body.

F] CoQ 10 Enzyme / Coenzyme Q 10

These are the nutrients that occur naturally in the body.

Uses Of CoQ 10 Enzyme

Cell Damage
It is used as an anti oxidant that protects cells from damage.

Metabolism
It plays an important part in metabolism.

Hypertension
There is evidence that the supplement of it can lower blood pressure.

Heart
It may improve symptoms in heart failure and other cardiac conditions but still a bit conflicting.

Memory
It can slow the progress of Alzheimer's disease.

Fertility
Co Q 10 has been used to treat infertile patients and low sperm count as an adjuvant therapy.

Migraines

It can be used as a preventive measure for avoiding migraine and headaches.

Deficiency

It is known that CoQ10 decreases with increasing age

Seizures	Intellectual Disability	Involuntary Muscle Contraction, [Dystonia]	Muscle Spasticity
Hearing Loss	Degeneration of Optic Nerve which Causes Loss of vision	In Infancy Severe Deficiency Leads To Brain Dysfunction and Muscle Weakness	By Late 60, It Causes Cerebella Ataxia, Problems with Coordination and Balance Due To Its Effect in the Brain

Foods with Co Q 10

Organ Meats	Heart, Liver, Kidney	Pork	Beef	Chicken
Trout	Herring	Mackrel	Sardine	Spinach
Cauliflower	Broccoli	Soy Beans	Lentils	Peanuts
Oranges	Strawberries	Sesame Seeds	Pistachios	

G] MSM / Methylsulfonyl Methane

A joint lubricant and wrinkle reducer

MSM is a sulphur chemical compound found in plants, animals and humans. It can be chemically made. It is a supplement very useful for our joints.

Uses of MSM / Methylsulfonyl Methane

Joints

It has a good anti inflammatory action which helps better mobilization of the joints, reducing pain and stiffness.

Cartilage

It inhibits the breakdown of cartilage.

Wrinkles

It is used as a topical solution to reduce wrinkles, eliminate stretch marks and treat minor cuts.

Exercise

It speeds up recovery after exercise.

Gut

It improves the leaky gut.

PMS

It reduces the PMS [Pre Menstrual Syndrome] symptoms.

Hair

It improves hair growth.

Deficiency of MSM / Methylsulfonyl Methane

Joint Inflammation @ pain	Chronic Fatigue, Muscle	Digestive Issues Decreases	Constipation Allergies

	Wasting	Immunity	

Foods with MSM / Methylsulphonly Methane

Coffee	Beer	Tea	Raw Milk	Whole Grains
Onions	Cabbage	Brussel Sprouts	Broccoli	Cauliflower
Grains	Apple	Tomatoes	Garlic	Raspberries

Caution

Those who are having allergy of sulphur should avoid taking it.

MSM is available in powder / capsule / or crystal form.

Dosage is 1000mg / day [RDA recommendation].

Chapter 6

Spices and Herbs

Cinnamon / Dalchini

Cinnamon is the dried brown, inner bark of the tree Cinnamomum zeylanicum. It is high in cinnamaldegyde which is thought to be responsible for health benefits.
In the ancient Egyptian times cinnamon was considered as a very valuable and rare spice. *It was given as a gift of devotion.* It is the most popular herb and has medicinal spice value.

Uses of Cinnamon

Powerful Antioxidant
Cinnamon has polyphenols [antioxidant] which helps fight against free radicals. It helps reduce inflammation.

Heart Protective
It may prevent against heart disease. Cinnamon helps in lowering LDL [bad cholesterol] and triglycerides.

Lowers Blood Sugar
It increases sensitivity to insulin thus helps lower blood pressure.

Weight Loss
Cinnamon also aids weight loss. It inhibits storage of fat for a longer time. My mom always advocated this use.

Prevention against Cancer
Cinnamon reduces cancer cell growth. The toxic effect of cinnamon help leads to death of cells.

Helps fighting against Diseases
Its potent content cinnamaldehyde helps the body fight against diseases.

Relieves Muscle Soreness
It is used to relieve mild PMS and allergic reactions.

Sugary Taste
Cinnamon has a natural sweet taste so adding to foods will require less sugar. Thus less sugar means weight loss.
To try: Try and use cinnamon in most of your foods. I use the jeera and cinnamon powder crushed together.

Turmeric / Haldi

Turmeric is the root of the plant Curcuma domestica. It has a deep yellow color and is commonly used in cooking. Everyone is well versed with turmeric, more so in this pandemic era of covid-19. Now they call it the 'The 'yellow milk'.

This is not new. Our ancestors made us drink turmeric milk, for cough, cold, and sore throat. Another use of it is, to heal the bleeding wounds especially on fingers and toes. It has antibacterial and haemostatic [controls bleeding] effect, meaning it will help fight infection and help clot the blood immediately.

I have personally used it and would advocate in emergency use to stop bleeding on fingers and toes only, and before you reach a doctor. It has many other uses too.

Uses of Turmeric

Anti Inflammatory
Putting turmeric on cuts and wounds helps early healing.

Homeostasis
It help in clotting of blood at the wound site especially toes and fingers.

Joints
The curcumin in turmeric acts as an anti inflammatory agent, reducing the swelling of the joints. This is beneficial for metabolic syndrome and obesity

Diabetes
Turmeric increases insulin sensitivity and reduces blood sugar.

Hypertensives
It suppresses adipogenesis and reduces blood pressure. It is particularly more beneficial when combined with piperine.

Brain Function
It improves brain function by helping in the regeneration of neurons. This prevents the degenerative process in the brain.

Food
Turmeric might be brain food.

Good for the Skin

It is used as a pack or gel on the face and makes the skin brighter and shiny.

Marriage Ceremony
It is an old tradition of using turmeric during wedding ceremonies. The turmeric is applied both to the bride and the bridegroom prior to the wedding. This is known to give a good skin texture.

Black Pepper/ Kali Mirch

Black pepper is the dried fruit of the plant Piper nigrum. White pepper is prepared by soaking black pepper and rubbing it to remove the outer coat.

The pungency of pepper is due to the resin Chavicine. The best way to take black pepper is freshly grounded pepper rather than add to cooked foods. But both are best.

Uses of Black Pepper

Digestion
It may help in digestion by increasing intestinal motility and thus preventing constipation.

Good for Health
Black pepper is used to treat cough and cold. Honey + black pepper, mixed together and then taken, is used for colds.

Detoxification
Pepper detoxifies your body thus preventing deformation of skin and thus helps reduce wrinkles.

Asafetida / Hing

Asafetida is the dried latex exuded from the rhizome or tap root of several species of ferula.
They are part of celery family. It contains an essential oil, gum and resin.
It is used for flavoring the food. It is used either as culinary or for medicinal purposes.
It is high in sulphur content, and thus has a pungent smell.
It is sometimes referred to as 'Stinking Gum'.

Uses of Asafetida
It adds flavor to dishes.
It is used as a preservative in pickles.
Has an anti inflammatory effect.
It acts as an anti oxidant, thus reduces your cell damage to free radicals.
Asafetida has been shown to contain high amounts of phenolic compounds, such as Tannin which is are known for their potent antioxidant effects.
It may help reduce symptoms of 'IBS' Irritable Bowel Syndrome.
Asafetida aids in digestion, relieves gas, and cures upset stomach.

Anti Cancer
The anti carcinogens effect occurs by preventing excess growth of the cells.
Special uses of Asafetida

Application of Asafetida in Infants
Asafetida is put around the umbilicus to relieve colicky pain.

Chest

Asafetida paste applied on chest to relieve asthma, bronchitis, cough, as it has antibacterial, anti viral and anti inflammatory effects.

Face

Asafetida applied on face increases the blood flow to the skin. Thus there is a glow on the skin, asafetida+ water= apply on face.

Bishops Weed / Carom/ Ajwain

Ajwain is derived from an herb plant that originated in our own very country.
It has a bitter and a pungent flavor somewhat like 'Oregano'.
It has been planted in my house and has been used frequently in place of oregano.

Uses of Bishops Weed / Ajwain

Pain

Chew bishops weed with a little salt twice a day. It greatly relieves your stomach pain, stimulates gastric juices and aids digestion. Thus relieves you of gas and bloated stomach. [This has been tried by me on advice of my mother for a year and was totally beneficial].

Digestion

It has a mild laxative effect by increasing the juices and aiding digestion.

It boosts the Immune System

The essential oil in Ajwain has antioxidant property which boosts the immune system and prevents free radicals.

Kidney

Ajwain / Bishop's weed help to prevent the formation of kidney stone.

Chest
It helps in asthma, bronchitis and cold. Just make a paste of Ajwain and jaggery and take it twice a day. It prevents nasal blockage and clears mucus easily.

Teeth and Ear
Used for ear and tooth ache. Just put a few drops of 'Ajwain Oil' in warm water and then gargle with it to relieve tooth ache.

Cumin / Jeera

The dry seeds, fruits of Cuminum cyminum contain thymol.
It is used as a regular ingredient for cooking. Used as a powder in many dishes and also to sprinkle in a glass of butter milk.
One can make tea with cumin seeds and sip it like the green tea

Uses of Cumin

Digestion
It helps improve digestion and relieves gas and bloating. Soak cumin at night in little water.
In the morning on empty stomach, chew the cumin seeds and drink the water.
It has a cooling effect and relieves acidity too. This trial has been done by me and obtained amazing results.

Anti Ageing Property

The Antioxidants [Apigenin and lutolin] in cumin help keep the tiny free radicals away that attack the healthy skin. The skin shows less ageing effects and remains healthy.

Roasted Cumin Powder

This roasted cumin powder is full Of 'Magnesium and Sodium.'

Cumin Oil

Cumin oil is a hypoglycemic agent and helps the diabetic in decreasing the blood sugar.

Helps Increase Hemoglobin

The cumin contains iron which helps to increase your hemoglobin [Hb].

Prevents Food Borne Disease

The antiviral and antibacterial properties of cumin help in fighting infection and food borne diseases.

Improves Bone Health

Regular intake of cumin helps the bone density, and the calcium in cumin helps the bones to be stronger.

It is a memory booster.

Children

It is also given to children, in doses of one or two teaspoon after each feed, to prevent intestinal colic.

Fenugreek / Methi Dana

This is one of the vey good seeds which are added as a flavoring agent to some of our cooking.

Soak fenugreek seeds overnight. One can chew or swallow the seeds with water.
Sprouted fenugreek seeds with papad make a delicious cuisine to eat.

Uses of Fenugreek Seeds

Hypertension
Fenugreek seeds have benefits of lowering blood sugar levels.

Hormone
Fenugreek is a medicinal plant popular for its purported effects on the hormone 'teststosterone'.

Appetite
It is a natural 'appetite suppressant' thus aids one to lose weight.

Hair
Beauty publications claim that fenugreek seeds are the secret to growing thick, shiny hair.

Digestion
Fenugreek water helps in flushing out the harmful toxins from your body and helps improving your bowel movement.

Milk Secretion
It helps increase milk production in breast feeding mothers.

Heart
It may also lower cholesterol.

Joints
It helps to lower joint inflammation.

It is an Old Age Therapy
Our parents and grandparents always advocated for healthy bones to take fenugreek seeds daily, chew or swallow.

Ginger / Adrak

The ginger plant (Zingiber officinale) is grown for its aromatic, pungent, and spicy rhizomes, which are often referred to as ginger roots.

The main active components in ginger are gingerols, which are responsible for its distinct fragrance and flavor. Gingerols are powerful anti-inflammatory compounds that can help alleviate the pain caused by arthritis. Studies have also shown that ginger helps boost the immune system, protect against colorectal cancer, and induce cell death in ovarian cancer.

Ginger is a daily ingredient in our foods and tea. In this Covid-19 ginger and lemon water is advocated. So ginger is famous, ginger tea, ginger powder and ginger in food

Uses of Ginger

Digestion
Ginger helps in digestion and relieves gas. Ginger stimulates the bile and promotes digestion and relieves 'flatulence'.

Liver
Also reduces the risk of liver ageing.

Throat
Helps in cold and cough - Ginger has known to increase blood circulation, thus help in relieving

cold and soothening the throat. *Hot ginger tea is advised.*

Acts as an Immunity Booster
It is now hyped in this Covid- 19. Ginger and lemon water is good. It also prevents the accumulation of the toxins in the body. It is an immunity booster which helps clean the lymphatic system.

Helps Reduce Inflammation
Ginger has the antioxidant and the anti inflammatory effect to reduce swelling.

Treats Severe Indigestion
Ginger helps in early emptying of the stomach and thus treats indigestion. One can chew ginger or take sips of ginger tea.

Reduces Premenstrual Cramps
Taking 1 gm of ginger orally daily for three days may help reduce menstrual pain.

Ginger is Bacteriocidial
It is bacteriocidal to the cellular structure and thus kills bacteria effectively.

Sperms
A Research has shown that ingesting 500 gm of ginger powder for 3 months, improves the sperm quality. Ginger protects the DNA.

Skin
Ginger acts as an anti-ageing agent and keeps the skin glowing.

Hair
Ginger helps in growth of hair and also reduces hair fall by increasing circulation in the scalp.

Beverages
It is utilized to produce aerated beverages such as ginger ale, ginger beer and ginger soda.

Garlic / Lasan

LET FOOD BE THY MEDICINE AND MEDICINE BE THY FOOD BY HIPPOCRATES [THE FATHER OF MEDICINE].

He used to prescribe garlic to treat a variety of medical conditions.
Garlic is obtained from the bulb of the plant *Allium sativum*.
Garlic warded off the evil eye, and was hung over doors to protect medieval occupants from evil, gave strength and courage to Greek athletes and warriors, protected maidens and pregnant ladies from evil nymphs, and was rubbed on door frames to keep out blood thirsty vampires. Today many shop keepers and households still follow these.
Garlic contains compounds with potential medicinal use.
Garlic is used in different cuisines to enhance the flavor.
It is used as a dip [chatni].
It can be chewed which is beneficial for heart health.
Scientist have researched and found out that most of its health benefits are due to the sulphur content Allicin. Garlic can be chopped, crushed or chewed. Alicin is one of the compounds that become instable when chopped or crushed.

Uses of Garlic

Garlic is low in calories. It is rich in manganese, Vit-B12, Vit-C, Selenium, fiber. It also contains calcium, copper, phosphorous, iron and Vit-B1.

Garlic can Combat Cold

A research has shown that consumption of garlic reduced the cold by 60%.

Blood Pressure

The active compounds in garlic can reduce blood pressure.

Heart Healthy

Garlic reduces cholesterol levels thus reducing the risk of heart diseases. It lowers LDL cholesterol. [Garlic supplements are available]. A dried garlic powder tablet is standardized to provide 0.6% allicin, when given as a standard dose of 300mg tablets three times a day to lower the cholesterol levels.

Gastro Intestinal

Allicin in garlic inhibits the growth of gram-positive and gram-negative bacteria. The natural form is used to suppress intestinal bacterial activity in diarrhea and flatulence.

Garlic Juice

Garlic juice diluted with water has sometimes been used as lotion for cleansing septic wounds.

Blood Clotting

Garlic inhibits platelet aggregation. The compound *Ajoene* has a anti platelet aggregation effect. Clotting time and fibrinolytic activity are considerably delayed after eating garlic.

Antioxidant
Garlic has antioxidants that may help prevent Alzheimer's and dementia. Here high doses of garlic are needed.

Life
It may play a role in extending life span.
Garlic may improve physical performance in animals.
Garlic helps detoxify the body by reducing the lead levels by 19%.

Bone Health
One study in menopausal women was done.
Garlic contains phyto estrogens.
Thus by taking 2gms of dry garlic extract daily will significantly decreases bone loss due to estrogen.

Green garlic in winter is very good.
Garlic is easy to include in your diet and changes the flavor of food to delicious.
Conclusion: Use of spices and herbs are essential in our daily life. Each one has its own specificity.

Summary: All the spices and herbs are essential for the body. So one must enjoy and take regularly

Chapter 7

Fruits - Their use in Diabetics

Seasonal fruits are best eaten as its richness of its nutrients and vitamins will help you a long way. Eat local as getting fruits from far will be less fresh.

Banana

This fruit is easily available, cheap, energetic and low in sugar. Banana has a rich source of potassium, magnesium, Vit-B6, Vit-C, iron, sugars and carbs. One average sized banana provides 100kcal.

Uses of Banana

Magnesium
It retains muscle power and prevents muscle cramps.

Potassium
It helps regulate blood pressure.

Carbohydrate
It gives instant energy.

Mild laxative
It aids in relieving constipation as it has a mild laxative effect.

Sleep
It helps to induce sleep by uplifting mood and acting as stomach filler.

Face
It has an antioxidant property and can be applied on the face and under eyes.

Diarrhea
Banana inhibits the growth of B-Coli by its release of butyric acid when taken in high quantities.

Wounds
Banana leaves can be steamed and are used for wound dressing.

Iron and Copper
Iron and Copper in banana helps prevent anemia. Copper assists in producing red blood cells. Thus it prevents anemia and improves blood circulation in the body.

Banana has a very soothing effect in case of sore throat. Bananas are a fruit for all ages. Banana is eaten as a fruit, in salads, in custard, as a vegetable, and raw bananas make lovely snack.

Apple

AN APPLE A DAY KEEPS THE DOCTOR AWAY

Apples are rich in iron, Vit-C and fiber and low in calories. It has antioxidants [polyphenols], trace of sodium, Vit-A, Vit-B1, Vit-B6 and folate, tannin, and pectin.

Uses of Apples
Apples are nutritious with 'no fat, no cholesterol'.

Weight

Apples are good way to keep your weight in place.

Diabetes
Eating apple is linked to lower the risk of diabetes.

Heart Friendly
Apples are good for the heart as it helps reduce cholesterol.

Iron
The iron content of apple raises hemoglobin and helps in preventing anemia.

Fiber
The fiber content increases intestinal motility and relieves constipation.

Antibacterial Property
Due to its bacteriocidal property it is useful in treatment of diarrhea. Apple helps to reduces arthritis and gout.

Cancer
It has substances that destroys viruses and have anti cancer properties.

Apple Cider Vinegar
The apples are crushed and exposed to yeast, which ferments the sugar and turns them into alcohol.
Next they add bacteria to further ferment the alcohol, turning into acetic acid which is the main active compound in vinegar.
The acetic acid gives the vinegar the sour taste and this is responsible for benefiting health.
It contains a substance called Mother, which consists of strands of protein enzymes, and

friendly bacteria that gives the product a murky appearance.

It also contains a small amount of potassium. This vinegar is heart healthy, having bacteriocidal property and aids in weight loss. It delays the emptying of the stomach.

Oranges

Our famous school song: Orange and Lemon so for a penny, all the school girls are so many, the grass are green and the rose is red, Remember me I am dead, dead, dead.

Saying this but the correct word for it is Staying Alive with Oranges.

Oranges are rich in Vit-C, folate, Vit-B, fiber, potassium, choline, beta carotene, citric acid, and are low in calories but are high acidic foods.

The urine can become alkaline if sufficient amount of oranges are taken as tannin is metabolized into carbonate.

Uses of Oranges

Heart Friendly
It helps lower blood cholesterol.

Antioxidant Property
The antioxidant content of oranges neutralizes the harmful radicals and prevents us from diseases.

Fiber
The fiber helps for better movement of the gut and thus helps in-digestion.

Potassium

It is needed for proper functioning of the nervous system. It is unsuitable in case of renal failure.

Lower Risk of Colon Cancer
It is linked with lower risk of cancer especially colon cancer, Oranges boosts our immune system.

Beta Carotene
Beta carotene action is to help smoothen the skin texture and decrease the effects of ageing.
Orange and its peel and are used in cakes and biscuits. The orange juices are yummy.

Beauty Packs
Oranges are used as an ingredient in various face packs.

Pineapple

It is a very juicy delicacy power packed with vitamins and minerals, and rich in bromelain and manganese.

Bromelain is also widely used as a commercial meat tenderizer due to its ability to break down tough proteins.

Pineapple is rich in Vit-C, manganese, copper, thiamin, folate, potassium, magnesium, niacin, pantothenic acid, riboflavin, iron, bromelain and manganese, also low in calories.

Also have traces of Vit-A, phosphorous, zinc and calcium.

Uses of Pineapple

Vit-C

It helps in growth and development and gives a healthy immune system.

Manganese
It aids growth, has an antioxidant property and also maintains a healthy metabolism.
Antioxidants in it are rich in flavonoids and phenolic acid. It helps your body to combat oxidative stress and inflammation.

Bromelain
It is an enzyme which helps in digestion, aids white blood cell function and it aids the death of cells in cancer.

Heart Friendly
It reduces clotting of blood, thus reduce the risk of heart disease.

Gums
The astringent in pineapple helps in strengthening of 'gums'.

Mangoes

I was always afraid to eat mangoes for fear of putting on weight. But I found out that eating mangoes is very good, and oh! If you do not over eat they are very healthy. I have abundant mangoes on my farm and now I relish and enjoy them as never before.

Mangoes are hot Latino super food / the king of fruits and have copper, folate, Vit-B6, Vit-E, Vit-B 5, Vit-K, niacin, potassium, riboflavin, manganese, thiamine and magnesium.

Small amounts of phosphorous, pantothenic acid, selenium, iron, low in calories with carbohydrates, proteins and less healthy fats.

Mangoes are delicious and can be eaten in various forms of pickles, as a fruit, dips, mango vegetable cuisine, milk shake, ice cream, etc. An average mango gives 50-100 kcal.

Mangoes are rich in Vit-A, Vit-C [25mg] and carotene [10,000 units/142 micromol]. *The ripening of mango increases the total amount of carotenoids. The beta carotene is 60 times higher than other fruits. Thus it may impart a yellow tinge to the skin if one ate too many mangoes.*

Antioxidant Property of mangoes

Mangoes contain Quercetin, Fisetin, Isoquercitrin, Astragalin, Gallic acid and Methyl Gallate. All this protects the body against breast cancer, colon cancer, prostate cancer and leukemia. It protects your cell against free radical damage and helps delay ageing.

Mangiferin [poluphenol] has gained the most interest and is sometimes called a *'super antioxidant'* since it is especially powerful.

Vit-C:
This is a water soluble vitamin and aids your immune system helps your body absorb iron and promotes growth and repair. It *improves skin's defenses and helps collagen formation, thus reducing wrinkles. The high amount of Vit-C helps in reducing inflammation and pain in the joints too. [My personal experience too].*

Vit- A

It is good for the eyes it contains the lutein and zeaxanthin. These accumulate in the retina of the eye the part that converts light into brain signals, so your brain can interpret what you are seeing in the retina. Lutein and zeaxanthin acts as a natural sun block. It protects the eye from harmful blue light, promotes hair growth and it protects skin from the sun.

Immune System
It helps to maintain a healthy immune system.

Magnesium and Potassium:
They help maintain a healthy pulse and keep your blood vessel relaxed, promoting lower blood pressure levels and healthy heart.

Digestion
Mangoes has an *enzyme called amylase* which breaks down large molecules of food, this helps the food to be absorbed better dietary fiber in the mangoes relieves constipation.

Remember
Mangoes are high in 'sugars', so eat in moderation.
It can also be used as a face mask.

Important Tip for cutting of fruits
Certain fruits should be cut horizontally or in round shape. The reason is that the fruit will taste more delicious as very little skin is around it. Try it with apple, guava, peaches, pear, etc.

Guava/Psidium Gujava

Guava *is also rich in Vit-C and the cheapest source of having vit-c. There is 212mg of Vit-C in/100gm of guava.*

Guava has the fat burning characteristic, along with the fiber content in it helps to reduce the belly fat naturally. It helps to regulate your metabolism. It's a win-win situation. Guava makes for a very filling snack and satisfies the appetite.

Guava Leaves

It contain very huge amount of Vit-C and dietary fiber, and can create smooth environment in intestines.

Guava Tea

Guava tea helps prevent complex carbs from turning into sugars. This helps the diabetics to reduce sugar. It also aids in weight loss.

Papaya

PAPAYA IS DELICIOUSLY SWEET WITH MUSKY UNDERTONES AND A SOFT BUTTER LIKE CONSISTENCY WAS REPUTABLY CALLED THE FRUIT OF THE ANGELS CHRISTOPHER COLUMBUS.

It contains Vit-C, folate, fiber, Vit-A, magnesium, copper, pantothenic acid and potassium. The unripe fruit is a good source of papain and is capable of digesting protein in all mediums, alkaline, acidic or neutral medium.

Eye health
It is loaded with Vit-A so good for eye health.

Anti Ageing
The carotenoids in papaya can neutralize free radicals.

Inflammation
The enzyme papin and chymopapain in papaya can decrease inflammation.
The protein dissolving papain is found in many exfoliating products.
These products help by removing dead skin of the clogged pores.

Food Use
Raw papaya is used in cooking to reduce the toughness in dals and meat.
Don't forget the papaya and the cucumber pack for the eyes to reduce dark circles.

Berries

They are low in sugar and carbohydrates and high in fiber and Vit-C, with manganese, folate, Vit-K, and copper.
All benefits are like the other fruits mentioned above.

Berries have low sugar content than other fruits. So people with diabetes can take them.
They are a more blood sugar forgiving fruit by Kimberly gomer a nutritional specialist.

Amla

They are rich in Vit-C. [600mg/100gm]

Grapes

Grapes are rich in calories and carbohydrates and low in Vit-C [3mg/100gm of Vit-C]

Pomegranate

The fountain of youth fruit

It is rich in tanin. The tanin acts on the intestines as an astringent and helps precipitate food.
It is the fountain of youth fruit and extremely good for the skin.

Important Tip
One must always eat fruits which are grown locally.

Eat all fruits which are available in your state. The fruits contain natural sugars i.e. fructose. Bananas are available all year round. Also have the seasonal fruits like mangoes, chiku, pomegranate, pineapple, sugarcane [the real detox]. All diabetics should eat fruits. It will help eventually control sugars. Fruits should be eaten daily.

Chapter 8

Vegetables

Spinach

Spinach is called a super food because of its high source of antioxidant and anti inflammatory properties. Spinach is rich in iron, Vit-A, Vit-K, Vit-C, potassium, magnesium carotene, manganese, little sugar and calcium, low in calories.

Uses of Spinach

Rich in Iron
The oxalates are rich in iron which helps carry oxygen to all parts of the body.

Potassium
This maintains the blood pressure levels.

Rich Source of Folate
This prevents the neurological defects in the new born, cellular function and tissue growth. The other content of spinach, Carotene, Vit-C and E. assist in reducing the risk of developing heart disease, cancer and cataract.

Eyes
Carotene of spinach helps prevent age related macular degeneration.

Vit-K
This helps in clotting of blood and the calcium strengthens the bones.

Important

Eating spinach raw or cooked is good, so don't fret.

Vegetarian times writes that folate, Vit-C, niacin, riboflavin, and potassium are more available in raw spinach. ,

Cooking increases the Vit-A, Vit-E, protein, fiber, zinc, thiamin, calcium, and iron. The other important carotenoids, such as beta-carotene, lutein, and zeaxanthin are also increased.

Important: The intake of Palak Paneer or Palak and curd decreases the absorption of calcium. So it is important to remember for people who are taking calcium.

Tomatoes

A study in agriculture and food chemistry showed that tomatoes release

Lycopene *[a cancer fighting antioxidant] When cooked,* but the raw tomatoes have equivalent benefits.

Tomatoes are rich in vitamins and minerals Vit-A, Vit-K, Vit-B1, B3, B5, b6, B7, Vit-C, Vit-E, folate, iron, potassium, magnesium, chromium, choline, zinc, phosphorous and quercetins.

The flavonoids [quercetin] and Lycopene have many protective effects on the body.

Vision

Lycopene also improves vision health, along with preventing night blindness.

Lycopene may help to prevent enlargement of prostate. It may also be responsible for blocking the production of hormones responsible for the growth of the prostate.

Tomatoes control the growth and the onset of cancer of prostate.

Beta-carotene, Vit-C, and Vit-E: They all help to lower risk of cataract, stroke and cancer.

Vit-K
It prevents formation of clots.
Sundried tomatoes and cherry tomatoes are equally good.

Fennel/ Sauf

This is a great digestive ingredient.

Uses of Fennel

Digestion
It helps indigestion, relieves constipation, bloating and gas.
It reduces the acid and thus acts as an antacid, i.e it relieves your acidity.
It helps purify blood, regulates blood pressure due to potassium, also helps to balance and prevents muscle cramps.
In infants the fennel seeds are added to gripe water thus easing the intestinal cramps.

Fennel acts like Oestrogen
Due to its estrogenic effect fennel has been used since a long time, to increase stimulation of milk, and for stimulating menstruation, it is an awesome coolant

Note

I have regularly take 1tsf fennel + 1tsf cumin, was soaked overnight in water. I drank the water on empty stomach and chewed the contents. [Advised by my mother]

It can be added to pickles, eaten as a mouth freshener, and add-ons to some vegetables and curries.

Fennel chewing gives a great relief in acidity, belching, gaseous distension and pain in stomach.

Coriander / Cilantro / Dhania

Coriander is rich in fiber, iron, magnesium, manganese, Vit-C, Vit-K, protein, phosphorus, potassium, thiamin, niacin and carotene.

Uses of Coriander

It reduces stomach spasm and relieves gas.

Coriander helps in the absorption of sugar and lowers the risk of insulin spike. Thus indirectly regulates blood sugar.

Cilantro oil, known as citronella, has anti microbial, antifungal and antioxidant property. This helps prevent mouth ulcers, clears skin dryness, fungal infection and eczema.

The uses of coriander are well known.

Basil / Tulsi /Holy Basil

It is a flavoring plant of the mint family [lamiaceae], grown for its aromatic leaves. Tulsi means the incomparable one or "the queen of plants." It is rich in Vit-C, Potassium, and Vit-A, calcium, iron, and Vit-B6, Vit-K, magnesium and omega-3 fatty acids. Tulsi has medicinal use. The leaves, stem and seeds all have medicinal value.

Uses of Tulsi/Basil

It increases immunity.

The Royal Melbourne University of Technology [Biology Section] says that the Tulsi oil at the concentration of 4.5% and 2.5% completely inhibited the growth of staphylococcus aureus and escherichia coli. They are severe hackling infections.

Tulsi / Basil Oil

The oil has anti microbial properties and is used to treat skin infections.

Tulsi / Basil Powder

It is used in herbal teas and cough mixtures. [Tulsi / Basil cough syrup].

The antioxidant [eugenol] treats the free radicals and reduces stress and heart disease.

It also lowers blood sugar, relaxes blood vessels, reduces memory loss associated with stress and ageing.

Inhalation of oils improves mental alertness.

Basil increases safety of foods when added to readymade manufactured foods.

Tulsi has astringent property which kills the bacteria, thus preventing cavity, plaques and bad odor of the mouth.

Important

One must tear the basil leaves for more flavors instead of cutting it. It is used in tomato / pesto sauces, vinegar. Also sprinkled on salads and tomatoes and used as an additive while making tea. The holy basil is used while offering puja to God on the food plate of fruits offered [bhog].

Cabbage

It is a rich source of sugar, iron, Vit-B6, thiamine, calcium, potassium, carbohydrates, antioxidants such as choline, beta-carotene, lutein and zaxanthin, flavonoids such as kaempterol, quercetin and Apigenin.
The red cabbage has more of amounts of these ingredients mentioned above.

Uses of Cabbage
Antioxidant
The sulphoraphene and kemferol helps to keep inflammation in check, as theses antioxidants reduce cell damage.

Fermented Cabbage
It helps to improve digestion and reduces constipation

Cabbage is great stomach filler, so helps to reduce weight.

The Vit-C helps to boost the immune system and a good skin healer.

Red Cabbage
It is a very powerful antioxidant, so reduces the risk of cancer, stroke and heart disease.

A research has shown that use of cabbage juice helps to treat acid peptic disease or peptic ulcers.

Caution

Consumption of cabbage in high amounts affects your thyroid substance called 'goitrogens'

Cabbage can inhibit iodine transport to the thyroid gland. [a process necessary for thyroid function]

Sweet Potato

The very name suggests sugar-and-starch. I give this root veggie two thumbs way up.

Uses of Sweet Potato
They are good source of Vit-C and A. One cup of baked sweet potato provides nearly half of your daily Vit-C + 400% of Vit-A.

Minerals
It provides a third of your needs of magnesium, that helps produce collagen and promote skin and bone health.

Antioxidant Powerhouse
Purple sweet potatoes give them their gorgeous hue has particularly potent antioxidant properties.

Anti-Inflammatory
Research done on animal has shown to reduce inflammation in brain tissue and nerve tissues, after purple sweet potato extract consumption.

Sweet potatoes do not cause blood sugar spike: The high fiber content makes them a slow burning starch—meaning they won't spike blood sugar and insulin levels.

One cup of baked potato provides 6gms of fiber.

Blood Pressure
One cup of baked sweet potato with skin provides 950mg of potassium. This amount of potassium is twice the amount in a medium banana.

Potassium essentially sweeps excess sodium and fluid out of the body, which reduces blood pressure and strain on the heart.

Weight Loss
About 12% of the starch in sweet potato is resistant starch, a filling fiber- like substance your body does not digest and absorb. Resistant starch also promotes the body to pump out more satiety-inducing hormones.

Try to
Eat the sweet potato baked with sprinkle of cinnamon and drizzled with maple syrup.

Smash sweet potatoes with oats and make a smoothie.

Add to a salad.

Use as a base for broth in soups.

Cucumber

Cucumbers are rich in water content and less calories.

It is a rich source of potassium, fiber, Vit-C, and small amounts of

Vit-K , magnesium, potassium, manganese and Vit-K.

Uses of Cucumber

It promotes hydration with its good water content [96%]

It is a powerful antioxidant which helps to reduce stroke, cancer, and heart disease.

Fiber content helps in regulating bowel movement and relieves constipation.

The sterols on cucumber help to fight the bad cholesterol.

Phytochemicals in cucumber have anti cancerous properties which boost the immune system by eliminating free radicals.

They are low calorie foods so can help to lose weight.

Cucumber reduces ageing effect. It hydrates the skin.

It is used as an eye pack, face pack and other cosmetics.

Carrots

Carrots are rich in Vit-A, Vit-K, beta-carotene, fiber, potassium and antioxidants.

Uses of Carrots
Carrots are weight loss friendly.

Vit-A
The Vit-A in carrots helps to improve eyesight.

In pregnancy women should be given Vit-A to prevent night blindness, but the blood pressure needs to be normal.

The fiber content impairs absorption of cholesterol from the gut and reduces heart disease.

Insoluble fiber in the carrots promotes regular bowel movement.

The carotene [antioxidant] is linked to reduce risk of cancer.

The biotin in carrots plays an important role in protein and fat metabolism.

My father drank carrot juice daily.

Chilly

Chilly has zero calories but packed with vitamins, Vit-A, Vit-C, iron, sodium, potassium, Vit-B6 and magnesium.

Uses of Chili
After eating chili your metabolism boosts up to 50% for three hours.

Has an antioxidant property and protects the body against free radicals.

Chili reduces blood cholesterol, triglycerides and platelet aggregation, thus heart friendly.

Capsaicin found in chili stimulates secretions which help to clear mucus and reduce congestion.

It also alters lipid catabolism and thermogenesis which helps against obesity.

Digestion: Chili increases the gastric juices and enables better digestion and destroys bacteria.

Mint

It is a food nutrient which converts them into energy. It is rich in sodium, potassium, fiber, Vit-A, Vit-C, Vit-B6, calcium, iron.

Uses of Mint
Mint stimulates the body to digest fat, thus helps to reduce weight, helps digestion, relieves constipation, smoothens gastric ulcers, and especially helpful in conditions with disease IBS [Irritable Bowel Syndrome].
It is a coolant and helps fight summer headaches.
The mint toothpaste [helps fight tooth decay], mint candy, mint gum, mint beauty products and mint oil.
Chewing mint leaves alleviates toothache.

The Vit-A in it promotes and maintains eye health.
Mint contains an antioxidant and anti-inflammatory agent called rosmarinic acid.
This acts as an anti allergic
Dips made out of mint taste delicious, and the water delicacy with other ingredients is awesome.
Mint lemonade, mint tea, and also added to juices and fruits.

Curry Leaves

They are rich in antioxidants, glycorides, alkaloids and phenolic compounds.
It also contains sodium, potassium, Vit-C, Vit-B6, Vit-A, and little of iron and magnesium.

Uses of Curry Leaves
They are rich in antioxidants. It keeps the body healthy, and reduces oxidative stress.
Rich in anti-inflammatory and anti bacterial properties which help in preventing diseases and thus promotes heart health.
It protects against neuro generative disease [but more research is needed]
The fibrous nature of *curry leaves* aids intestinal motility, and protects liver from stress or damage.
The antibacterial, antifungal and antioxidant properties help the skin infections like acne, skin allergies, and fungal infections

Word

It is an old age tradition or custom to bathe with neem leaves. Neem soaps are also available for skin.

Yogurt

It is used daily in most of the households having tangy taste. It is rich in zinc, sodium, potassium, protein, calcium, cobalamin, b6, selenium and magnesium.

Uses of Yogurt
It makes the bones and teeth healthy.
It contains a lot of calcium which helps maintain it.
The protein in yogurt is high and thus causes fullness of stomach and controls the appetite.
Restores gut health. Yogurt contains probiotics which may boost digestive health. Reducing bloating, diarrhea and constipation
Live yogurt restores gut health and it is a proven fact.
Immune system: The magnesium, zinc and selenium play a role in maintaining the immune system.
Skin and health hair: Zinc in yogurt helps the skin to be shiny. Hair when washed with yogurt strengthens the roots and makes it shiny, in south it is a tradition.
Yogurt increases the good HDL cholesterol which protects the heart.
The lactobacillus and acidophilus in it decreases the low density lipoprotein [LDL] the bad cholesterol. *This also prevents the occurrence of gasto-enteritis and vaginal thrush, pepti ulcer*

and urinary tract infections. Good to maintain vaginal flora.

Weight Management
Yogurt is high in proteins along with calcium to increase the levels of appetite reducing hormones like PPY & CCK. So this may help weight management.

Beware
The readymade yogurts of different types contain a lot of sugars, thus read the labels properly, hence homemade yogurts are best.

Coconut

Coconut water and grated coconut is very good for health, try adding to your foods. It has good amount of potassium.

Skin and Hair
It enhances the skin texture. It helps to improve the moisture content of dry skin.

Coconut oil can also protect against hair damage.

Weight Watchers
It helps to reduce weight. The fatty acid in it helps to burn fat. It has the shorter chain fatty acids.

Brain
It helps in preventing Alzheimer's.

It provides quick energy to the body.

Heart Health

Kitavan people in Papua New Guinea ate a lot of coconut, alongside tubers, fruit and fish. These community ends up with not ending in stroke or heart disease.

Anti Microbial Effects

Lauric acid makes up about 50% of the fatty acid in coconut oil.

When you take coconut oil the lauric acid forms a substance called monolaurin.

Both lauric acid and monolaurin can kill harmful pathogens.

Mouth Wash

There is evidence that using coconut oil as a mouth wash, a process called oil pulling benefits oral hygiene

Good Cholesterol

The natural saturated fats help to increase the good cholesterol HDL.

It is also known to reduce the bad cholesterol LDL.

The Bottom Line

The oil derived from coconuts has a number of emerging effects for your body health.

Tips

Try including coconut in your foods as an when you can.

Add it to your snacks, salad and vegetables.

Drink coconut water.

One can also drink edible coconut oil which is available in the market.

Summary
One should eat all vegetables variant in colors.

Palak has extremely good effect. Sweet potato is rich in fibre and Vit-C.

All fruits which are seasonal and round the year available must be eaten.

Coconut is an essential to eat and not to forget pomegranate the fountain of youth.

Chapter 9

Nuts

OH NUTS \ I AM TOTALLY CRAZY ABOUT YOU.
NU+S ABOUT + YOU.

SOME NUTS ARE HARD TO CRACK,
BUT AIN'T NO NUT EVER GOES UNCRACKED
KEEP TRYING
BY SOHAN SAHU.

God Nuts Are All The Sweeter When Shared With Friends.

Almonds

They are low in calories and have low glycemic index.
They are rich in Phyto nutrients, Calcium, Fats, Vit-E, Amino acids, iron, manganese, magnesium and proteins.
Raw Almonds /Almond Butter: Which is the latest?

Low Glycemic Index
Almonds are good choice for people on low carbohydrate diet.

Fat
The fat in almonds is high but it is in form of monosaturated fat which is protective to heart and also lowers the lipids.

Phyto Nutrients
Sterol and Flavonoids are heart healthy.

Proteins
Almonds have both essential and non essential amino acid, which is a beneficiary nutrient.

Vit-E
It confers anti oxidant properties and supports immune function

Bone Health
Calcium in almonds maintains bones and teeth healthy.

Iron
The iron helps to build hemoglobin and hence more oxygenation to the blood.

Reduced risk of Diabetes
The magnesium and manganese play a role in reducing the sugars.
I love eating my Almonds daily.

Walnuts

LIFE IS A WALNUT - SHORT AND HARD TO CRACK.
BUT ONCE YOU KNOW THE SECRET TO CRACK IT.
IT'S ALL SWEET AND BEAUTIFUL AND GROSS.

Walnuts are rich in Omega-3 fats and contain higher amounts of antioxidants and fiber.

They are low in carbohydrates but high in Fats.

Walnuts are Energy dense and High in Calories.

Uses of Walnuts
Walnut being rich in omega 3 fatty acid and antioxidants, prevent the growth of cancer cells, including Pancreatic, Prostate and Breast cancer.

It adds shine and strength to the skin and hair.

Heart Protective
The ALA [Alpha Linolenic Acid] and Linolenic acid, decreases cholesterol levels and prevents heart disease.

It acts as an anti-inflammatory too.

Remember
Walnuts should be chewed well to get the oils.

Cashews

The unsalted dry / roasted cashews are low in Sugars, and rich in Plant Proteins and healthy Fats.

They are rich in copper, magnesium, iron, phosphorous, thiamine, selenium, Vit-K and Vit-B6.

Uses of Cashews
They are a good source of energy.
Cashews are rich in unsaturated fats and thus linked to a lower risk of premature deaths.

Healthy Brain
The significant amount of copper in cashews is responsible for good healthy brain.

Less Oxidative Damage
The Polyphenoids and carotenoids present in them reduce the oxidative stress.

Weight Loss
Cashews appear to provide fewer calories than once thought. Their rich fiber and protein content can help reduce hunger and increase fullness in the stomach.

A research says that Type 2 diabetes persons who consumed their 10% of calories from cashews had lower LDL [bad cholesterol] to HDL [Good Cholesterol] ratios, then those who did not eat cashews at all.

So enjoy eating your cashews without any worries.

Flax Seed / Sesame Seeds

One of the best foods which are richest in calcium and also have *Phyto estrogenic effects on the body*.

Flax seed improves the estrogen level in the body, thus eliminating mood swings, hot flushes and irritability.

The Ligans, Phytochemicals and omega-3 reduce inflammation, give better skin, aids reducing wrinkles and add shine to the hair.

The Ligans also help to reduce plaque formation in the arteries.

The manganese in it is good for bones and healthy blood flow.

Thus decreases anemia and prevents osteoporosis. It is the richest source of calcium

They are rich in both soluble and non soluble Fiber, regulating blood sugar levels of Diabetics.
I enjoy eating sesame seeds. All time is good time for me to eat them.

Chia Seeds

They are currently one of the world's most popular health foods.
Chia seed is full of fiber; therefore the digestible net carbohydrates are very less.

Peanuts

Peanuts are technically legumes, but tend to be prepared and consumed like nuts.

It is rich in fiber, magnesium, Vit-E, minerals, antioxidants, fats, proteins, carbs, sodium, potassium

Peanut butter is in use since long. It's never too early for Peanut butter.

This is one of the healthiest of snack and fills the stomach well

A handful of peanuts roasted without oil and salt are sometimes a good snack to have.

Grains

Grains are essentially sugar with enough Opiods to make them addictive. Come one and all and join the chain of addiction here.

Oats

Oats are healthy grains and are gluten free.

They are rich in carbohydrates, fiber [Beta Glucan], manganese, phosphorous, magnesium, copper, iron, zinc, folate, Vit-B1, B5 and with small amounts of Vit B6 and B3.

Lowers Blood Pressure Levels
Oats has a unique group of antioxidant called 'Avenanthramide'.

They help in lowering blood pressure levels by increasing production of nitric oxide.

This gas molecule helps dilatation of blood vessel and lead to better blood flow.

Anti-inflammatory and Anti-Itching:. The Avenanthramide in oats reduces inflammation and itching.

Helps Lower Blood Sugar and Cholesterol
The Beta - Glucan in it reduces blood sugar and bad LDL cholesterol.

Weight Loss
Oats gives a filling of fullness very easily due to beta-glean and promotes healthy gut bacteria.

Eating oats gives fewer calories, and delays the time it takes for your stomach to empty.

B-Glucan promotes the release of peptides YY & PYY, a hormone produced in the gut in response to eating. This is a satiety hormone.

Finely Ground Oats for Skin
Colloidal oat meal [finely ground oats] is used for dry and itchy skin. It is used a face scrub too.

May Help Relieve Constipation
The soluble and insoluble fiber in it helps better intestinal motility and treats constipation.

Summary
Besides fruits, vegetables, grains, herbs, spices even vitamins, minerals, calcium and sunlight are equivalently important.

It's a combo package that will lighten you, drive you, strive you to the person you want to be.

Kriss Carr says:
For nearly a decade now,
I've been teaching others
How to thrive by filling their bodies

WITH ENERGIZING VITAMINS, NUTRIENTS, MINERALS, ANTIOXIDANTS AND PHYTO NUTRIENTS. NOT A DAY GOES BY WHEN SOMEONE DOESN'T WRITE ME TO SAY,: THANKS I FEEL BETTER NOW, TOO" THOSE LETTERS FROM MY READERS ARE MY DIGITAL CARDINALS.

Chapter 10

The Hunger Inhibitor

A] Leptin

Leptin is a hormone made by the adipose cells and enterocytes in the small intestine.

Importance of Leptin
Leptin helps to regulate energy balance by inhibiting hunger. This in turn diminishes fat storage. Leptin does not affect the food intake from meal to meal. It acts to alter food intake and control energy expenditure over a period of time. Leptin signals the brain to the hypothalamus for this action.

Action of Leptin to Reduce Hunger
Food - Leptin - travels to brain - signals hypothalamus and controls appetite centre - binds with neuropeptide 'y' - turns of appetite switch -fullness from food.

Leptin Foods

Avoid High Calorie Foods	Get Enough Fiber	Eat Vegetables Fruits	Avoid Sugar and Sugary Drink, limit fructose
Take Proteins	Meat, Turkey Chicken,	Adequate Sleep, reduce stress	High Intensity Interval Training Exercises

Leptin Resistance

It occurs with high levels of leptin. The brain is starved. Resulting is obese body.

This is what obesity is, It is brain starvation. Leptin is fat related hormone. It has shown to produce weight loss in animals by decreasing appetite and increasing metabolism.

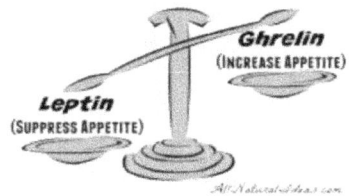

B] Grehlin

Hunger hormone

This is the hunger hormone. It stimulates appetite, thus increases food intake and this invariably leads to fat storage.

It is an amino acid secreted in the stomach and the pancreas. It influences growth hormone secretion.

It creates connection between the gastrointestinal system and the pituitary.

So food intake - hypothalamus appetite centre stimulation - turns on neuropeptide - leads to increased appetite.

Increase in Grehlin Hormone

Fasting	Low protein intake	Taking high foods in fats, sugar	Lack of sleep, avoid sleeping during, after meals
		Take supplements	Of multivitamin, calcium and

How to Decrease Grehlin

Good protein intake	Last meal at 8pm	Eating at 4-5 hour intervals	Good sleep
	Avoid sugar	Avoid refined foods	Avoid readymade foods

Summary: learn to control your leptin the hunger reducer and grehlin the hunger stimulator. Keep the balance between the two. Sleep and stress disturbs this balance

Adiponectin

Fat Burning Hormone & Regulates Glucose Levels

It regulates glucose levels and is a protein hormone. It has a close connection to insulin sensitivity and diabetes.

Action of Adiponectin
It causes increased breakdown of Fat into fatty acids and Inhibits glucose production from the liver. It has anti inflammatory effects on the cell lining the walls of blood vessels, hence increased levels of Adiponectin, and decreased risk of heart disease. *It is reduced if one has more visceral fat, so this is a fat burning hormone.*

Foods To Boost Your Fat Burning Hormone
The researchers have found that intake of Monosaturated fats, e.g. Fish oil, will boost your Adiponectin levels by 14 to 16%, other foods are avocado, nuts, olives, Olive oil, sunflower oil, 4 capsules of linoleic acid.

Fill up with Fiber

Adding fiber to the diet will increase the Adiponectin levels as much as 115%. It also stabilizes the glucose level and reduces the Glycemic impact of meals. Thus it improves insulin sensitivity.

35gms of fiber / day divided in four meals goes a great way to improve its levels.

Important
Adiponectin has tremendous influence on your fat loss and hormonal balance is profound.

Exercise
Moderate exercises 3-4 times a week is necessary.

Don't kick off your coffee habit. Coffee before a workout or early in the day will go a long way to burn fat. This will increase the Adiponectin levels and reduction in Pro-inflammatory cytokines which could boost weight loss and reduce inflammation levels.

Top Up the Turmeric
Take 2 capsules of turmeric half hour before meals.

Red Wine
Resveratrol found in wine stimulates Adiponectin. Both are equally important as they display anti ageing properties, anti inflammatory effect and as an agent to decrease obesity.

Consume your Carbohydrate at Dinner

A research study in 2012 at the Herbew University Of Jerusalem showed that carbohydrates eaten at dinner, rather than taken during the day seems to benefit people suffering from severe and morbid obesity.

The Iranian Journal of Diabetes and Obesity [2012] said that Zinc supplement helps in decreasing obesity. Zinc=50mg daily. Take tablet Zinc Citrate or Zinc Picolinate 50mg/day, for a maximum period of 12 weeks. Then one should switch over to multivitamin containing zinc.

So Folks Great Weight Loss

Hey Doc, find a new invention by applying a gastric band a meal which is complete with fiber, proteins and complex carbohydrates.
Doctor do a new invention
Just by thinking or dreaming
You become a desirable woman
One gastric band on
The magic band turns you
To a thin slim sexy you. Dr Maya

CCK

CCK is produced by lining of duodenum. It acts on two types of receptors found in the gut and released by neurons in the brain. It helps in digestion and appetite. Contracts gall bladder. Releases stored bile in the intestine.
Inhibits gastric emptying –meaning it delays the foods to go down from the stomach and acts both on the proximal stomach and the pylorus.

Foods to Increase Gastric Emptying

One Must Eat Low Fat, Fiber Foods
Chew Your Food Thoroughly
Avoid Carbonated Drinks, Alcohol, Beverages
Eating Fats Will Trigger Release of CCK
Take plenty of proteins every meal
Eat soft well cooked meal

One Must Take 5-6 Meals A Day

PYY

Pure younger and younger

Appetite Reducer Hormone

This is a hormone that decreases your appetite. It reduces food intake and reduces obesity. Once you eat the stomach has a sense of fullness.

Beware

Over eating cause Dilatation of Your Stomach on left side. It also bloats up and shapes up on one side like a balloon.

Cycle of action of PYY is: you eat food, then peptide yy is released, it circulates in the blood, binds to receptors in brain, decreases appetite, thus making your stomach full.

Foods to Increase PYY

Low Intake of	No Refined	No	No	Plenty of

Carbohydrates	Foods	Sugar	Carbonated Drinks	Proteins from Animals, Plants
Take More Foods Rich in Fiber				

GLP

It is a Glucagon like peptide that is secreted in the small intestine. It increases insulin release, delays digestion of food and makes you feel fuller.

Summary

Adiponectin is your fat burning hormone.
And thus helps in reducing obesity.

CCK will improve digestion and give a feeling of fullness in the stomach.

PYY decreases your appetite.

GLP increases insulin release and delays digestion of food to cause fullness in the stomach.
So everyone remember and incur it in your daily habits.

DR. MAYA MODI HAS A SPECIAL MESSAGE

I HAVE COME WITH A SPECIAL MESSAGE
AN OPEN FORUM WITH HIDDEN MESSAGES
CONNECT TO YOUR INNER SELF

FOR A NEWER BETTER SELF
CHANGE THE OLD SYSTEM OF SELF
ADAPT TO THIS NEW SYSTEM OF SELF

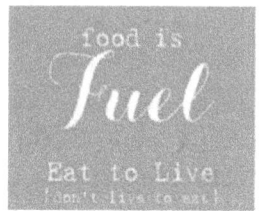

Remember nothing is difficult. It is a question of making a list and forming a habit.

To eat is a necessity but to eat intelligently is an art.

We all eat, and it would be a sad waste of opportunity to eat badly.
So grab your opportunities, and don't miss out on it.

WILLIAM SHAKESPEARE:
　　THIS ABOVE ALL, THINE OWN SELF BE TRUE
　　　IT MUST FOLLOW AS THE NIGHT THE DAY
THOUST CANST BE FALSE TO YOURSELF

Part 2

Chapter 11

Importance of Foods

For Different Parts of your Body

MAIMONIDES SAYS:
"NO DISEASE THAT CAN BE TREATED BY DIET SHOULD BE TREATED BY ANY OTHER MEANS

We all make good choices. Everyone likes good cars, good clothes, good body, and good house.

So why not invest in good foods.

Learn the Art of Living Healthy, from Eating the Right Foods.

Thus find a path to a Healthier and Happy Life.

Learn the ins and outs that are needed from here.

Carve a path to help yourself through foods for different parts of the body.

I will tell you the different foods for your body.

So then start making a plan how to utilize it. If need take help of a doctor or a nutritionist. The benefits are ample and time tested.

Beauty comes from within

K

A] Foods for Skin and Over All Health

BEAUTIFUL SKIN REQUIRES COMMITMENT, NOT A MIRACLE
[ERNO LAZLO]

The earlier you take action the better it is.
Beautiful glowing skin starts with how we eat, but these anti ageing foods can also help with more than that. When we pack our diet with vibrant foods loaded with antioxidants, healthy fats, water, essential nutrients, our body will show its appreciation through its largest organ, the skin.

After all the skin is often the 1ˢᵗ part of our body to show trouble. We need to take a further look at what fueling us, rather than use creams, serums and masks. Thus take plenty of veggies and fruits.

Cleopatra's beauty secrets are still relevant today. Cleopatra has always been regarded as one of the world's most beautiful woman with a flawless skin. The word of her stunning looks and beautiful skin spread from one generation to the next. The ancient Egyptians were famous for their beauty rituals even 5000 years ago. Cleopatra was the queen of beauty and so many innovations were done by her. The Egyptian queen's beauty techniques were so progressive that many of secrets are still relevant today.

Sea salts: Cleopatra realized the healing properties of one Dead Sea salts. She was famous for using them for its natural healing properties. It's unknown whether she fully realized the full range of benefits that salts gave the skin. By replacing the essential minerals, but they were a key part of her beauty routine. *Sea salt was used as a scrub.*

Kohl the Egyptians really embraced this makeup. Kohl was the basis of one of the most famous inventions, the Eyeliner. Cleopatra used to create a famous cat eye that she has owned for 5000 years. Kohl wasn't only beneficial as a beauty product. It protected the eye from the sun, while also protecting from infections.

Milk and honey face mask was used by Cleopatra. It had a hydrating moisturizer effect on the skin.

Skin tips by Cleopatra: It is said that for soft and glowing skin Cleopatra the Egyptian beauty used to mix milk of a young donkey with fresh honey and almond oil.

Tip: Mix a cup of honey with 3 cups of milk and add 5 tablespoon of almond oil. Now add this mixture into your bath and get that gentle soft skin.

Sea salt scrubs a natural and a wonderful skincare regime. They can help exfoliate, clean and moisturize your body. Cleopatra used this natural scrub to exfoliate her body and face.

Tip: Take two tablespoons of sea salt and mix it with three tablespoons of thick cream. Now gently rub your face and body with it in circular motions and leave it on your skin for at least 5 minutes. Later rinse with rose water. Rose water is easily available in the market and has many benefits for all skin types from cleaning to cleansing and toning. It refreshes, revitalizes and adds glow to the skin. Rose water also has anti-inflammatory properties that can help reduce the redness of irritated skin. Cleopatra used to wipe her face with rose.

Tip: Just take some cotton dipped in rose water and wipe your face, morning and evening for a beautiful glowing skin.

Cleopatra face cream consists of beeswax, rose water, essential oils and aloe Vera juices.

Tip: Take beeswax and almond oil and make a liquid of it. Now add Aloe Vera juice, rose water and essential oil into the substance and mixed thoroughly. Once it is melted completely, allow it to cool down and store the cream in your refrigerator. You can use the 20 wax cream whenever you want to.

Natural shampoo: Cleopatra used egg to wash her hair, a natural shampoo to make her hair soft and beautiful.

Tip: Take 3 eggs with water in a bowl, mix it and wash your hair with this chemical free natural shampoo.

1] Cleopatra loved to use honey on her face due to its antibacterial properties.

2] She washed her face many times a day. She used oil and added lime to it.

3] She used to rinse her face with apple cider vinegar

4 The other things used were ginger antimony, calamine, onions, goose fat, turpentine, etc.

These were some of the numerous skincare products used in Queen Cleopatra's skin care regime.

Cleopatra used rose water to make the pimple marks disappear.

Cleopatra used Henna or a mixture of Juniper berries, oil and two unidentified plants to dye her hair.

Besides these, olive oil was used to enrich the hair texture.

She added Dead Sea salt to her bath with essential oils and aromatic flowers. This would relieve stress and get a glowing skin. She used milk for bathing. The Vit-A and E in milk acted as an antiseptic.

If she can do it we can also make efforts to get a beautiful skin.

Foods for Skin

1] Watercress:

It is rich in calcium, potassium, manganese phosphorous, iodine, Vit-A, Vit-C, Vit-K, B1 and B2.

It is rich in water and hydrates your skin and an internal skin antiseptic, also increases circulation to deliver minerals to all cells of the body. It enhances oxygenation of skin. The antioxidants Vit-C and A, neutralizes free radicals. Thus helps to keep fine lines and wrinkles at bay.

Other effects of watercress are it boosts your immunity, good for digestion of food, can act as a diuretic so less fluid retention in the body, can increase your energy. It supports the Thyroid function due to its iodine content.

Add water cress to your salads and sandwiches.

2] Red Bell Pepper

They are rich in Vit-C and Antioxidants

Benefits for Skin and Overall Health

Bell peppers are good for production of collagen. It contains a powerful antioxidant called carotenoids which are plant pigments, red, yellow, orange peppers. *So protects the skin from sun damage, pollution and environmental toxin.*

You can eat it raw with humus, add to a salad or sandwich or can make a vegetable and savor it.

3] Papaya

Papaya is rich in antioxidants, Vitamins and Minerals. It contains Vit-A, Vit-C, Vit-K and E and calcium.

Papaya contains and Enzyme Papain. This *gives an additional anti-ageing and anti inflammatory effect.*

Papaya is found in many of the creams, face mask and scrubs.

Try and eat papaya drizzled with a bit of lime it tastes very delicious. One can make papaya mask at home.

4] Blueberries

They are rich in Vit-A, Vit-C and has the age *defying antioxidant called Anthocyanins.*

Benefits of Blueberries

The antioxidant protects the skin from damage to sun, stress and pollution. *It prevents collagen loss and has mild anti-inflammatory effects.* They are also low in sugars.

To Try

Use this low sugar berries as a fruit or a morning smoothie but it may not be available everywhere.

5] Broccoli

Broccoli is power packed with Vit-C and Vit-K, fiber, folate, Lutein and variety of antioxidants.

Benefits of Broccoli

The lutein in it is linked to the preservation of brain function. Calcium is needed for bone health.

The Vit-C is the main protein in skin that gives its strength and elasticity.

To Try

One can eat lightly boiled broccoli or add to salads, broccoli almond soup and pesto sauces can be made

6] Spinach

Spinach is spiced up with Vit-A, Vit-C, Vit-E, and Vit-K, magnesium, hydrating and power packed with antioxidant and has plant based haem iron.

Benefits of Spinach

It is hydrating, increases oxygenation and replenishes the entire body. Vit-C enhances collagen formation to keep skin firm and smooth. The Vit-A in it gives strong, shiny hair. It also has an anti-inflammatory effect.

To Try

Spinach used to make a smoothie, alone or with other ingredients. Can make vegetable or use it to make pasta.

7] Nuts

There's a great metaphor that one of my doctors uses: If a fish is swimming in a dirty tank and it gets sick, do you take it to the vet and amputate the fin? No, you clean the water. So, I cleaned up my system. By eating organic raw greens, nuts and healthy fats, I am flooding my body with enzymes, vitamins and oxygen.

Walnuts

Walnuts strengthen the skin cell membrane, protects against sun damage. It preserves the natural oils to give the skin a beautiful glow. Walnuts reduce risk of heart disease.

Almond

Almonds help repair the skin, retains moisture, and protects skin from damaging ultra violet rays. They have the potential to prevent cognitive decline in older adults.

Pistachios Reduce risk of type 2 Diabetes.

To Try
It is very essential to chew the walnuts well for its oils to be effective. Almonds eaten soaked are good and filling to the stomach. Can eat as a snack or add on to salads, cakes, biscuits, etc.

8] Avocado
Avocado is rich in Vit-A, Vit-C, Vit-K, and Vit-E, Vit-B.

Benefits of Avocado
Avocados promotes smooth supple skin, it has anti-inflammatory effects. The Vit-A helps shed dead skin and gives a gorgeous glow to the skin. The carotenoids help to protect against skin cancers and prevent damage from sun.

To Try
Avocado can be used instead of butter, in a sandwich. Can make a smoothie, as a fruit or add to a salad.
One can use it as a face mask to fight inflammation. It reduces redness and helps prevent wrinkles.

9] Sweet Potato
Sweet potatoes are rich in Vit-A, Vit-C, Vit-E and antioxidants.

Benefits Of Sweet Potato
Sweet potato helps restore skin Elasticity, promotes skin turn over, gives a youthful look,

softens the texture of skin, protects the skin from free radicals and keeps the complexion radiant.

To Try
You can eat it boiled, baked or add to vegetable.

10] Pomegranate Seeds
Pomegranate is used as a Healing Medicinal Fruit.

Benefits of Pomegranate
Pomegranate has a variety of antioxidants which prevents damage from free radicals. It reduces inflammation in our body.

Pomegranate also contains a compound called 'punicatagins' which may help preserve collagen in skin. It also contains estrogen and progesterone.

To Try
Eat it as a fruit, make a juice, and can sprinkle it on salads and other dishes.
Research has shown that a compound called 'Urolithin - a' which is produced when Pomegranate interacts with gut bacteria.

This may rejuvenate Mitochondria and has been seen to reverse muscle ageing in rat studies.

Summary for Skin and over-all Health
Fruits and nuts and spinach, bell peppers, sweet potatoes avocado, pomegranate, blueberries, papaya and watercress should be a part of your daily routine plate for skin and overall health.

B] Foods to Increase Collagen

I remember when I was starting out as a young actress, thinking, Oh my God, "I have the fattest face" Now I look at those pictures and I think, 'So much collagen!'

Collagen maintains elasticity of skin, reducing ageing effects and decreases joint pains.

Benefits Of Collagen

It Improves Skin	Reduces Hair Loss	Restores Collagen of the Face, making it tighter	Builds Stronger Muscles
Promotes Bone Health	Strengthens Your Immune System	Healthy For the Heart	Detoxifies the Body
Better joints	Improves sleep	Has antioxidant property	Less wrinkles

You can supplement your diet with foods and vitamins that boost collagen production in your body.

Foods for Collagen

Fish with Skin	Chicken, Beef	Bone Broth Oysters	Egg Whites
Tomatoes	Bell Peppers, Red, Yellow	Beans	Spinach & Sweet potato
Pomegranate	Sun Dried Tomatoes	Kale, avocado	Citrus Fruits
	Foods Amino Acids	Zinc Found in Oysters, Beef, Crab	Copper Foods Found In Organ Meats Cocoa

		zinc foods	Powder, Mushrooms
Garlic	Collard greens	Cashews	Berries
Antioxidant Rich Foods. Collagen Fillers Available, Also PRP, Plasma Rich Platelet Treatment	Salmon with Lemon, Sweet Potato Kale And Avocado Gives Great Anti Aging Meal	Chicken Taco with A Scoop Of Collagen Peptide Sweet Potato, Onion, Avocado, Lime, Makes True Anti Aging Meal	Caesar Salad with More Nutrient Dense Leafy Greens, Kale, Spinach, Or Add Nuts, Seeds For Some Crunch - To Avoid- Bread
Quinoa, Red Wine Vinaigrette, Black Beans, Cocoa Powder, Vanilla Extract, Dijon Mustard	Worcestershire Sauce, Tortillas, Sprouted Whole Grain Bread, Collagen Peptides	Salt, Pepper, Cumin, Smoked Paprika, Chili Powder, Cinnamon, Olive Oil	Tomatoes, Eggplant, Legumes, Asparagus, Turmeric, Ginger

Glycine found in gelatin, chicken skin, pork, shallots, red onions, scallions, lime, banana, chicken breast, salmon, almond milk, flax milk, parmesan cheese, plain goat milk yogurt. Super foods like Maca, Spirulina Acai

Hyaluronic acid is a great way to hydrate and reduce wrinkles. It is a cosmetic cream. It works great, and is something to use after derma rolling to speed up the healing process. It is available in capsule form also.

Supplement with antioxidants, amino acids, minerals, proteins, copper, zinc, chlorophyll and Vit-C are to be taken.

Some actresses do go for excess energy face lift. It is a spiritual way to tighten the face of the skin with Rekki. Some of them use fillers.

Summary
Supplements can be taken on advice of a doctor.

The skin of the fish is a rich source of "type 1 collagen", which accounts for the majority of the collagen in the skin.

Drink plenty of water and sleep well.

Skin and Collagen - *A Special Mention*

Skin is composed of collagen, elastin and connective tissue. For repairing the skin certain nutrients are essential to keep it supple, shiny and hydrated. So repair, rehydrate and revitalize.

Essentials for the skin

1] Cell walls of the skin are made up of lecithin and lipids. Puffy eyes are the result of wasted water build up.

2] Lipids

Here the primary most essential lipid is EFA [essential fatty acids]. EFA have the ability to attract this wasted water from the cells and infuse it inside your cells. *They are essential and our body is not able to produce it. Essential fatty acids are available in cold water fish, nuts, seeds, and vegetable oil.*

3] Lecithin

Lecithin is there in the cell walls of the skin. A diet rich in lecithin and EFA will help and rebuild your cell walls and keep the water inside your cells in their original place.

4] Dermis of the Skin

Dermis is made of collagen and elastin. It contains amino acids and the rest of the matrix is made up of GAGs including for example Hyaluronic acid. Glucosamine is needed for building up the Hyaluronic acid.

Glucosamine is an essential nutrient vital for the joints and is used in the treatment of arthritis. Glucosamine helps to repair the weakened tissues and helps reverse the debilating pain of arthritis. By supplementing the body with these nutrients the weak tissues in your body becomes firm as years go by. *Thus helps to decrease the sags, dimples and help as fillers.*

5] Now is the time to repair the connective tissue. Connective tissue is made up of matrix or substances called glycosaminoglycans or GAGs. To repair this matrix the body needs amino acids, glucosamine which are the building blocks of collagen. The amino acids help keep blood vessels firm and in shape.

6] How to prevent deterioration of blood vessels and the creation of spider veins. Like the skin the blood vessel is made up of collagen connective tissue and elastin. A diet rich in nutrients will help to fill the blood vessel and keep it strong. It is not always for the body to get all nutrients from foods.

7] Connective tissue is made up of chondroitin, dermatan and mostly Hyaluronic acid. These nutrients are converted in the presence of glucosamine. The body does produce glucosamine but not in sufficient amount to replenish all the connective tissues. Hence glucosamine supplements are to be taken.

Tablet glucosamine in dosage of 1000-2000mg/day this will reinforce the connective tissue with GAGs.
Hyaluronic acid is the nutrient which keeps the skin joints and connective tissue hydrated. Thus as you age there is less production of Hyaluronic acid which causes dryness in the joints and wrinkly skin.

8] Amino Acids
Amino acids are the essential which build and repair the collagen and elastin in blood vessels.
This can be obtained from sufficient proteins from our foods. They are nuts, seeds, beans, whole grains, vegetables, fruits and Goji berries. Goji berries are not available easily. The other foods are tofu skinless white meat and fish rich in Omega3.

9] Essential Amino Acids
The connective tissue of the blood vessels is repaired by essential amino acids. They are found in nuts, seeds, flax seeds, sesame seeds, walnuts and cold water fish. Those who are not fish eaters need to take supplements.

Fish oil tablet = 100mg/day, flaxseed oil tablet=1000mg/day
DHA supplement=100-300mg/day. One can take sesame seeds too

Essential Amino Acids

The essential amino acids are lysine, tryptophan, theonine, leucine, histidine, methionine and phenylalanine.

Non essential amino acids

The non essential amino acids are alanine, cysteine, arginine, aspartic acid, asparagines, proline and tyrosine.

Along with it take vitamins, niacin and pantothenic acid, cobalamin, pyridoxine, riboflavin, thiamine, folic acid and biotin. According to RDA allowances one need to take a multivitamin and b-complex tablets.

Along with it minerals are also required like magnesium, iron, zinc, copper, manganese, iodine, chromium and selenium. It is better to take iron and zinc separately. One must understand that all the nutrients are not available in the multivitamin tablet. Thus it is essential to take different types of multivitamins. Along with it one must take supplements and foods rich in essential fatty acids, vitamins, amino acids and glucosamine. This will help to fill up collagen and elastin fibers and reduce your skin wrinkles.

The foods are milk, eggs, cheese, nuts, wheat, meat, poultry and leafy greens. Soy foods are known to contain good amount of essential amino acids.

10] Dermis of the Skin

To keep the dermis of the skin supple and smooth you need to replace the nutrients, that the damage cells have lost. Essential fatty acids are needed to rebuild your cell wall and attract the lost water back into your cells. This will hydrate the skin throughout the body.

Along with essential fatty acids, lecithin and lipids rich foods are to be taken.

One can take supplements of lecithin tablet 2000 to 4000 milligram of Soya lecithin granules or 1 large egg does the trick.

Sources of Lecithin:

Lecithin sources are eggs, spinach, lettuce, cauliflower, peanuts, peanut butter, tofu, Soya lecithin granules, oranges, apples and potatoes. Along with the foods also take essential fatty acids, vitamins, lecithin, glucosamine, b-complex, minerals and trace elements.

11] Exfoliation of Skin

This is a daily ritual for me. I use milk on my skin which has good exfoliation effect and keeps my skin smooth and supple and glowing.

The other exfoliating agents are glycolic acid which is in sugarcane and salicylic acid. To use this do consult your doctor. The other essential things is brushing off your skin and moisturizing your skin. One must use moisturizers which have Vit-C, zinc, glycerin Vit-E, Hyaluronic acid, Alovera, pomegranate extract, salicylic acid or malic acid.

12] Antioxidants are Essential

Polyphenols are family of antioxidants. They are found in found in tea, grapes, red wine, pomegranate, raspberries, strawberries, nuts, whole grain, cereals, vegetables, colored fruits, soybeans, Vit-C, Vit-E, Vit-A, CoQ10 enzyme and anti-inflammatory foods.

Alpha Linolenic Acid Sources Of Foods
Lettuce, broccoli, spinach, lima beans, peas and split beans and gamma linolenic acid foods

Summary for Skin and Collagen

A] Supplements and trace elements

They are primrose oil, black currant oil glucosamine, lecithin, antioxidants, essential amino acids, Vit-B and minerals.

B] Fats of 3-4 servings

They are omega3, olive oil, nuts, and flaxseed oil.

C] Proteins of 4-6 servings

They are eggs, yogurt, cheese, chicken, and fish.

D] Whole grains of 4-8 serving

E] Fruits of 3 or more serving and vegetables 4 or more servings.

F] Sleep 8hours a day.

G] Take adequate water. Eight glasses per day.

H] Do facial exercises.

I] reduce your stress.

J] Don't forget your Vit-C.

My tricks of good healthy skin:

I have a very good smooth skin. The first thing is good nutrition and plenty of water. Milk does wonders to your skin. I daily apply milk on my face, neck and hands since many years. i do circular movements on the face and eyes too. It moisturizes your skin and it give a little bit of peeling effect. This way you're dead skin is removed

The other trick I have learned for the skin is very simple and effective to use. I moisturize my whole body daily after my bath with Alovera cream. I finish my bath, towel dry and then immediately I apply the cream all over the body. Many people are habituated in cleaning the bathroom, but I would say no to it. Either you finish the work before or leave it for doing it later. Immediately meaning,—absolutely immediately. The aloe Vera gel is not to be used as it would shrink your skin.

On applying the cream, the absorption of it is quick as the body is slightly wet and the vessels are opened up.

Besides this to keep the wrinkles at bay I do facial exercise daily. The right time for me is mainly when I am driving and making monkey faces in the car. People just stare at me I just wink and say hi to them

These are the facial exercises, no specific time is needed. I believe I can do it anywhere and if someone laughs, its fine, just avoid it [ki farak phenda] meaning who cares

I also do tapping off my face. I start from the chin upwards to the face on to the forehead. I do the round, upward circular stroke.

Using a soft brush on the skin is always also a good idea because this would increase the blood flow to the face

It is always best to keep the face clean.

I learnt to cure my pimples myself after trying many medicines.

I did treat many patients for pimples. I would only see them after they were tired with all the super specialists.

All the people are very fond of the parlor to do get their facials done. I for one have had very less facial in my life. I feel it gives a very typical look to your face. I have more trust on the dermatologist and the plastic surgeon. I would take advice from them. I prefer to do the chemical peeling of the face with a solution which keeps all the pores clean and peels of the dead skin. This I learnt from the plastic surgeon Dr Umesh Shah. This is a very helpful technique and gives better results than even a facial.

Supplements:

I do take supplements off and on. I have the habit of using different brands of medicines. This is because all the supplements are not available in one tablet.

I use collagen and glucosamine powder once a week.

The other supplement I am very happy with is tablet Centrum and tablets Vigorex.

These are multivitamin tablets and are very good for the skin and overall health.

One does develop B complex deficiency very often. I for one always know the signs and symptoms. In order to avoid this deficiency I take B complex injections every 4 months

The foods are plenty Pomegranate, banana, papaya, avocado, eggs and nuts a very healthy for the skin.

The skin will glow when you shine when your inner side is happy. Good sleep is very important. If you sleep well it shows on the face. So enjoy your beauty sleep. Besides this exercise plays a vital role.

C] Foods to Reduce Inflammation

There are many types, but these are the main ones. Inflammation can be anywhere in the body and the diseases are many. Arthritis is one of them where there is swelling of the joints and severe unbearable pain.

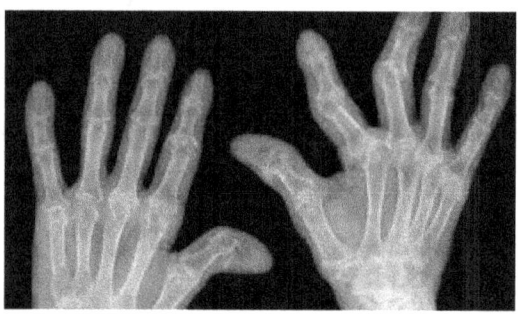

Do you want this Arthritis?

Foods to Reduce Inflammation

Fatty fish, such as Salmon, mackerel, sardines and trout helps to reduce inflammation. The American heart institute recommends at least 2 Servings of fatty fish / week. They are high in omega-3 fatty acid. This has beneficial effect by reducing inflammation, pain and morning stiffness. Antioxidants can be considered as anti-inflammatory as they prevent the free radical damage.

Other foods

Garlic, ginger	Spinach	Walnuts	Berries, cherry juice
Grapes	Broccoli	Olive oil	Tarts

Millet	Brown rice	Quinoa	Juice of cucumber
Cauliflower	Beetroot, celery	Beans and peas	

Medicines and application of gels are prescribed too. One thing I found very useful is moringa leaves and drumstick soup. This reduces inflammation slowly and steadily. Allantoin, Alovera, chamomile, arnica and zinc are helpful.

Moringa Leaves to Reduce Inflammation

Moringa which is grown everywhere and is easily available, yet we underestimate its power. I too started its use just few years back. These leaves have a great benefit for Arthritis. I have personally experienced the use and the joy I obtained from the relief of pain on my left ring finger.

How to Consume Moringa Leaves

The capsule and powder form are available, but not preferable. Only fresh leaves or dried leaves must be used. You can dry moringa leaves at home and then crush them in a mixer and store it in glass bottle.

How to Use Moringa Leaves

Take 10 to 15 leaves of moringa with little water, add lime juice [1/2 a lime] and add few drops of honey. Crush in the mixer and drink it daily. One will start getting results in one to two months. Don't take more than the leaves as mentioned.

Benefits of Moringa leaves

The benefits are countless. It reduces arthritis and osteoarthritis pain and swelling. Helps relieve constipation by increasing intestinal motility. Protects and nourishes hair and skin.

The bones become healthier. It also treats mood swings, reduces body fluids, lowers sugar, improves circulation and is a super food to improve sexual function in both men and women. It detoxifies the body, protects the liver, and prevents hair and cell damage. It balances the body's cortisol levels and reduces stress. In menopausal women it improves hot flushes and treats sleep disorders.

Moringa is a Medicinal Plant

All parts of the moringa tree are useful. The drumsticks are good in taste too. Our reverend Honorable Prime Minister Shree Narendra Modi has drumstick parathas, like stuffed bread.

Moringa leaves are caffeine free. The Vit-C is 7 times higher than Oranges. Vit-K is 15 times more than banana. It is useful overall. The moringa leaves are from the drumstick plant.

Satvik Healing for Arthritis

I have seen a video of a young girl hardly 17 years who had given up all hopes of walking or doing anything as she had severe arthritis. She was depressed, could not move, needed help from other people for her daily activities. Then she did Satvik healing. After following this satvik healing religiously she is able to run and walk and do her daily chores.

What to do in Satvik Healing

The first and foremost is she went out of the house to a garden.

Here she inhaled fresh air and enjoyed the rays of the sunlight. So she got Vit-D and breathing in this fresh air changed her life completely.

So exercising in natural environment and in this atmosphere filled her body with oxygen and vitamin-D.

We know that oxygen is very healthy and will not allow the disease to survive. This improved her blood circulation too. Initially she started with whatever stretching exercise she could do under supervision of a trainer. She was taught different techniques of breathing. The exposure to the sun helped her to strengthen her bones. Sunshine is God's gift that she was able to live a life that is free of disease. She did not give up and once she started noticing that her range of movement increased, she stuck to the plan.

Like magic, her body started healing and there were changes in her and her whole body in 3-6 months. Her hemoglobin started to increase, the inflammation decreased which can be seen in her blood reports. She visualized a beautiful picture of her Future. She knew the pain in her body is temporary and it will not last. She will be not dependent on painkillers or Steroids. This is a daily routine for her. She said to herself, be patient, there are no leaps but only hopes.

She was full of gratitude in every single breath she took. Don't procrastinate. She says take action right now, and magic of light will illuminate you. She walked down the road with a big smile.

So what is one waiting for? Don't think anything else and just follow the program. It is a must for people who are suffering.

Along with the outdoor exercises she followed a diet plan. There was no caffeine intake. She took a glass of cucumber juice+ celery + spinach + seasonal fruits daily in the morning.

Breakfast would be of fruits papaya/pomegranate/musk melon
Lunch would be one grain with lots of vegetables [pumpkin, carrots, beet root, beans or peas].along with millet or brown rice or quinoa.

Dinner would be stir fry vegetables [cauliflower with beans along with peas.] soup, and some raw salad.

She was told not to take any sugars, refined foods and processed foods. This difference turned her into a new person.

The solution to biggest health problem is simple. We just have to align ourselves back with nature.

Summary
Don't miss out on the outdoor activities basking in the sunlight. Simple as it seems but useful more than ever.

D] Foods for the Eyes - *A Better Sight*

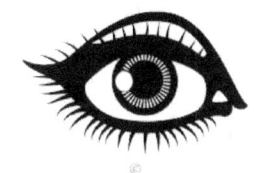

WHAT WE SEE DEPENDS ON
WHAT WE LOOK FOR

JOHN LUBBOCK

The eyes need Vit-A, Carotenoids, Lutein, and Zeaxanthin.

Vit-A

Carrots help in night vision and ability to adjust in the dark. It is high in beta-carotene and is an essential precursor for Vit-A.

Raw carrot / juice	Humus of carrots	Pumpkin, sweet potato	Cantaloupe
Citrus fruits, peaches, tangerines, water lemon	Lemons	Derbanana has carotenoids	Low fat milk is a good source of Riboflavin, reduce risk of cataracts.
Apricots	Asparagus	Guava	Kale
Mangoes	Mustard	Collard greens	Nectarines
Pink grape fruit	Broccoli	Squash	Garlic, onions are antioxidants for lens of the eye

| Tomatoes | Beet | Beef | Liver |

So production of glutathione is increased which is useful for the lens of the eyes.

Sunglasses

Use sunglasses when out in the sun and take breaks from digital device. This will make your eyes less tired.

Lutein and Zeaxanthin for the Eyes

They are essential to prevent or slow down macular degeneration of the eye. It can occur by excessive exposure to UV light especially high energy visible light [HEV] zeaxanthin is found in the macula of the eye and has a darker pigmentation, which in turn helps to keep harmful Blue light from reaching the Retina; it serves as a natural Sun block.

Foods for Lutein and Zeaxanthin

Egg yolk	Kiwi	Spinach	Peas, kale
Drum sticks	Carrots	Zucchini	
Orange juice, squash	Sweet potatoes	Grapes, mango	Lutein 10mg/day zeaxanthin is 2mg/day is the recommended dosage
Apricots, cantaloupe	Lettuce, broccoli	No smoking	Capsule intake of Lutein, zeaxanthin recommended

Important

Lutein and zeaxanthin reduce the risk of eye diseases, cataracts and age related Macular degeneration. A number of studies have shown that lutein decreases the oxidative stress to liver and eyes.

Omega3 Fatty Acids

It helps to reduce dryness of eyes and may prevent it too.

Salmon, tuna	Hemp seeds	Mackerel	Sardines
Walnuts, tofu	Chia Seeds	Brussel Sprouts	Algal Oil
Sesame Seeds	Flax Seeds	Perila Oil, canola oil	Flaxseed Oil

Summary for Eyes

Remember Vit-A, Vit-C, omega-3, minerals and beta carotene is important. Enjoy carrots, spinach, eggs, banana, mangoes pumpkin Chia seeds, tofu and other foods.

Important for Eyes

Do not forget to do the eye exercises. Start with rolling of the eyes round and round, and then blink with them. Keeping the head steady look up with the eyes and down, then look to right and look to left. I do them and are very helpful.

E] Foods for the Hair - *Strong Hair*

> *I LOVE MY HAIR BECAUSE*
> *IT'S A REFLECTION OF ME*
> *AND ME IS BEAUTIFUL*
>   *BY [BETTYDAIN]*

The condition of our hair is dependent on environment, foods we eat, water, hair washing, oiling of hair and combing of hair.

Foods for the Hair

Eggs: They are abundant in	Blueberries, tomatoes act as

protein, biotin.	antioxidant
Spinach for the production of sebum or oil in the scalp	Blueberries promotes production of collagen
Yogurt gives minerals, vitamins	Sweet potato forms the hair structure, Helps sebum formation
Meat has iron and it helps in making hair cell protein	Walnuts, selenium will protect the hair from sun damage
Biotin, Vit--E, copper, omega-3 strengthens the hair follicles	The tablets of these are available across the counter
Carrots, prunes, green peas, shrimps, oats, low dairy products prevents thinning of hair, corrects dryness	Kiwi juice stimulates hair growth. Lettuce + Honey + cucumber + lemon juice is good.
Walnuts + raisin + dried parsley + ginger + honey is good	Beet root + carrot + apple + honey is also good
Banana + spinach + honey juice	Fruits: Oranges prevents hair fall
Guava prevents hair breakage	Peach keeps the scalp healthy
Lime stimulates hair growth	Apple will increase volume of the hair
Banana strengthens the hair	Strawberries prevents hair loss
Papaya reduces thinning of hair	Tomatoes, Salmon are rich in omega-3

Alovera

Alovera is a proteolytic enzyme that heals and Repairs damaged cells in the scalp. It boosts hair growth and improves health of hair follicle and promotes regrowth of hair.

Oiling the Hair

Oiling of hair is like greasing your engine of the car for better output. Coconut oil is a good option for hair. It keeps the hair shiny, soft, and nourishes the hair follicles.

Summary

You should oil your hair on regular basis. Intake of iron and manganese foods, greens and fruits are necessary'. Age related hair loss is always there. One can apply Minoxidil solution or can opt for plasma rich platelet treatment.

My tricks: Comb your hair in a good manner. Take small portion of hair, twist it and start coming from the tip of the hair towards the scalp. The foods mentioned above and eggs do wonders to the hair.

F] Foods for Gums & Teeth – *Healthy and Shiny*

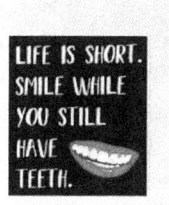

There are many diseases of the teeth and the gums. You should brush your teeth twice a day and try using different tooth pastes.

Fiber Rich Foods

They keep your teeth and gums clean and healthy says the American Dental Association.

Calcium Rich Foods for Teeth and Gums

Cheese	Low Fat Milk	Fat Free Milk, Saliva Maker
Walnuts,	Canned Salmon,	Black Tea Or Coffee

Almonds	meats	
Foods With Fluoride	Sugarless Chewing Gum	Spinach, celery, Carrots and beans

Vitamins for the Teeth and Gums

Iron and Vit-C are essential for oral and periodontal health.

Take Vit-D and calcium to make the teeth strong and along with it take vitamins with potassium, phosphorous, Vit-K and Vit-A.

Fluoride for Teeth and Gums: Fluoride, one of the dentist favorites. It can strengthen and re-mineralize damaged Enamel, making it more resistant to decay.

Fluoride is added to drinking water, tooth paste and mouth washes.

Foods with Fluoride for Teeth and Gums

Spinach	Raisins, grapes	Black tea, as it is made in water, water contains iodine	White wine has twice the amount of iodine then red wine
Hash or baked potatoes - more fluoride than fried chips	Black tea can stain your mouth more than coffee	Gargling of the mouth with normal water after eating chocolates or taking sugar	Oral hygiene is to be maintained by brushing twice a day

Summary

You must rinse your mouth thoroughly. It is necessary to use different tooth pastes. Brush your teeth morning and evening. Take foods given above and Vit-A, Vit-E, Vit-D, Vit-K, Vit-C, and calcium intake is essential.

Use of turmeric, salt or soda bicarbonate to clean your teeth once a while is good idea. I do follow this regime.

Fracture of teeth occurs easily. If you need implant, then get it done early, don't wait. This is because there is structural change of the face.

Calcium and Vit-D3 are an essential part. Just try keeping this in mind. There shall also be difference in chewing.

G] Foods for Mouth Ulcers

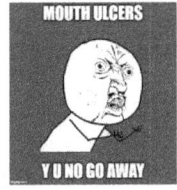

Having ulcers in the mouth are a great torture.

Causes of Mouth Ulcers

Indigestion	Constipation	Lack of folic acid	Lack of B12
Lack of iron, lack of zinc	Eating too much sugars	Bacteria in the mouth [helicobacter pylori] or one is taking antibiotics	Diabetes, Gastric band operation

Foods to Heal Ulcers of the Mouth

Vegetables, grains	Papaya	Potato, pumpkin,	Honey, yogurt, milk
Boiled eggs	Cottage cheese	Non spicy foods	Orange juice

| Cooked cereals, soups | Avoid vegetarian foods to increase the levels of acidity in the body | Apply a paste of baking soda with water on the sores | Avoid salty foods |

Medicines for Ulcers

You need many vitamins and diet changes relieve constipation and treat any disease you have. Essential for the ulcers is Vit-B12, Vit-E (600 I. U) , Folic acid 10mg twice a day, Vit A (10,000 I. U), Vit-C, Zinc 50 mg, Germanium 60mg thrice a day, Digestive enzymes, Antifungal and antibiotics. Apple cider vinegar gargles are good and can also gargle with Alovera mouth wash. Try using Alovera tooth paste.

These ulcers may be bad and it may take a while to heal them. Many a time a biopsy is required to rule out dangerous pathology.

Summary for Ulcers

Apple cider vinegar gargles should be done. Rinse mouth properly. Brush your teeth properly. Take Vit-A, Vit-B12, Vit-E, zinc, germanium, anti fungal and antibiotics.

Chapter 12

STELLA PAYTON SAYS
"PEOPLE TAKE OWNERSHIP OF
SICKNESS AND DISEASE BY SAYING THINGS LIKE
MY HIGH BLOOD PRESSURE,
MY DIABETES, MY HEART DISEASE,
MY DEPRESSION. MY! MY! MY!"

DON'T OWN IT BECAUSE IT DOES NOT BELONG TO YOU

These are the biggest concerns of life.

The diseases are exceeding tenfold due to fast foods, sedentary lifestyle and glued to ones seat for work. Let's do Bhangra with the Dhol.

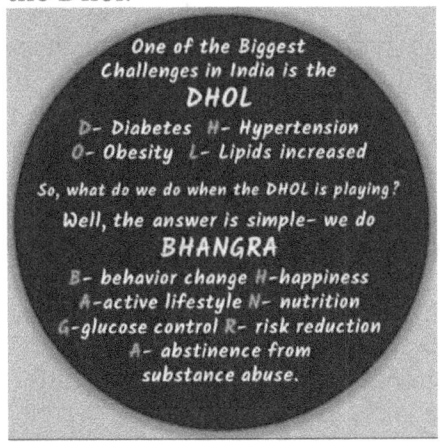

A] Diabetes

Diabetes **Mellitus** comes from two words. Diabetes, Greek for to pass through or Siphon, and Mellitus is Latin for "Honey or Sweet".

My brother Harry developed diabetes at the age of 30 years. Harry's father, sister and other brother were also diabetic. So Harry thought that it is genetic. I have seen Harry suffer and also has a few complications.
This is when I started to think and find ways for myself so as to not end up being diabetic.

Diabetes is characterized by chronically elevated blood sugar in your body. This is because your pancreas is not making enough Insulin or your body becomes resistant to Insulin. Insulin is a hormone that keeps your blood sugar in check.
If too much of Insulin it can come through the kidneys and spill into your urine.
Type 2 Diabetes is mainly due to high fat / high calorie diet and poor life style. It is called as Black Death of the twenty first century. Due to Type 2 Diabetes various complications occur such as diabetic neuropathy, vision loss, kidney failure and even deaths occur every year.

The carbohydrates you eat are broken down into glucose [the fuel for the body]. Glucose requires insulin to get them into the cells from the blood stream. So the accumulation of fats inside the cells of your muscles and liver interferes with the action of the insulin.

When glucose is denied entry into your muscles [primary consumer of such fuel] the sugar levels rise damaging the blood vessels.

The fat inside this muscle can either come from the fat you eat or from your body fat.

Thus prevention, treatment and reversal of Type2 Diabetes is dependent on diet and lifestyle changes

Good **News**

Type 2 Diabetes is preventable, treatable, and often reversible.

Insulin Resistance

The marker of Type2 Diabetes is insulin resistance. As previously said blood sugar to enter the cell requires Insulin, hence when the cells become resistant and do not respond to insulin, which leads to availability of sugars in the blood stream. They do not metabolize and don't burn glucose.

When you consume lots of carbohydrates, you get lethargic afterwards. It is a sign that you are developing insulin resistance. Should probably check fasting blood sugar in the morning [fasting blood sugar] 110mg, and then be cautious for you are developing insulin resistance. FBS of 80mg is normal.

What to do with Diabetes

Changes in Lifestyle for Type 2 Diabetes.

1] The recommended lifestyle interventions include: Taking two and a half hours each week of moderate intensity physical activity or one hour and 15 minutes of high intensity exercise.

2] Losing weight gradually to achieve a healthy body mass index.

3] Replacing refined carbohydrates with wholegrain foods and increase intake of vegetables and other foods high in dietary fiber

4] Reducing the amount of saturated fat in the diet

5] Physical activity

6] Nice recommend taking either 2 ½ hours of moderate intensity physical activity or 1 ¼ hours of intense exercise.

Moderate Intensity Physical Activities for Diabetics

A] Brisk walking.

B] Cycling on relatively flat terrain.

C] Water aerobics.

D] Hiking.

E] Rollerblading

F] Using a manual lawnmower.

Vigorous Physical Activities for Diabetics

A] Jogging.

B] Swimming

C] Cycling either rapidly or over steep terrain.

D] Football.

E] Gymnastics.

F] Skipping.

Some people may be able to be referred for structured or supervised exercise sessions.

Weight Loss for Diabetics
Guideline issued by NICE recommend those that are overweight aim to lose weight gradually until a healthy BMI is achieved.

Healthy BMI Range
A healthy BMI ranges between 18.5 and 24.9 or between 18.5 and 22.9 for people of South Asian descent.
For those with a BMI above the healthy range, NICE recommends aiming to achieve weight loss gradually, with a target to reduce weight by 5 to 10% over a period of a year.

Weight loss can help to reduce the risk of developing diabetes and can enable people with existing pre-diabetes or type 2 Diabetes to control the blood glucose levels.

If you have a BMI of over 30, your GP may refer you to take part in a structured weight loss program. People unable to achieve weight loss via lifestyle changes may be prescribed a weight loss pill called Orlistat.

Dietary Changes for Diabetics

The general dietary advice from NICE to reduce risk of type 2 diabetes is to decrease intakes of fat and increase intake of dietary fiber.

People who are currently overweight are advised to eat smaller portions to consume fewer calories. NICE recommend achieving a higher amount of fiber in the diet by including wholegrain foods in the diet and consuming more: Vegetables, fruits, beans and lentils.

Fat Intake

The advice on fat is to reduce overall fat intake, and particularly to reduce intake of saturated fat as found in chips, crisps, pastries, biscuits and samosas.

Lean Meats

One must choose lean meats, such as skinless chicken and turkey helps to cut down on saturated fat. It is recommended to eat less processed meats. Grilling and steaming of the food will cut down on fat intake in comparison with cooking methods involving frying or roasting.

Fruits

All diabetics must have all the fruits. Try and eat seasonal fruits. There is nothing as saying no to a fruit. All the fruits contain fructose which is well utilized in the diabetics. Eat local fruits, as they are healthier. Eat local, think Global.

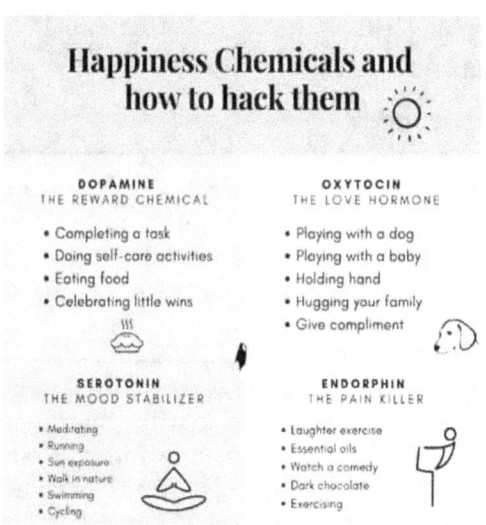

The human body undergoes a number of changes; stress hormones can activate the immune system. Non-crucial bodily functions such as digestion, growth and repair are slowed due to constant stress can make blood glucose control very difficult, particularly if an individual is unaware of when they are getting stress.

Constant stress can make blood glucose control very difficult, particularly if an individual is unaware of when they are getting stressed. Stress management techniques such as mindfulness are a simple non-toxic way to control stress related blood sugar changes.

Additionally, by reducing stress levels, chances of developing diabetes related complications such as heart disease, stroke, hypertension and mental health conditions including depression and anxiety.

Glycemic Index

The glycemic index is more important for the diabetics. The carbohydrates written on the labels include sugars and starch in the food. The fiber content of the food is not included here because fiber is not broken down during digestion. Therefore total carbohydrates include sugar, starch and fiber in the food.

This means that foods made with sugar and flour tend to have Higher Glycemic Index, than then the one made with whole grains intact. Thus their fiber content has been "Ripped off" during processing and thus left with more sugar and starch content than fiber.

Just watch out and be careful especially for diabetes, heart disease, metabolic syndrome and obesity.

Glycemic Index of Foods

Oats 1 cup=58, White Rice one cup=64, Brown Rice 1 cup=55, Lentils 1 cup=29, Chickpeas 1 cup=31, Mango 1 cup= 51, White Bread 1 slice= 70, Whole Wheat Bread or Chapatti 1 cup= 62. Popcorn 1 cup=72, Rajma 1 cup=28, Apple 1 medium=38, Mango 1 cup=51, Orange juice 1 cup=57, low fat Paneer 150 gram=35, Boiled Potato 1 cup=51, Kohler one cup-63, Soya milk 1 cup=44, Plain Yoghurt 1 cup=36, Whole Milk 1 cup=40, Ladies Finger 1 cup=20, Jamun 1 cup=10, Watermelon 1 cup=55, Frozen Peas half Cup=50.

Portion Sizes

Reducing portion sizes will also help to lower calorie intake. The Diet Plate is an excellent solution if you are looking to control your calorie intake fight or flee the threat that is instigating the threat response. Constant stress can make blood glucose control very difficult, particularly if an individual is unaware of when they are getting stressed.

Stress management techniques such as mindfulness, is a simple non-toxic way to control stress related blood sugar changes. Additionally, by reducing stress levels, chances of developing diabetes related complications such as heart disease, stroke, hypertension and mental health conditions including depression and anxiety, reduce dramatically.

Summary of Diabetes

Keep a regular check on your blood sugar. Walk, exercise, do portion control of foods and take less of carbohydrates and fats in your diet. One should avoid sugar and high glycemic index foods. Eat all types and varieties of fruits.

Sugars

The table has turned upside down from cholesterol to sugars. The newer studies have shown that sugar is the killer which becomes a stepping stone to your grave. We know that ultimately everyone dies but sugar is the causative factor for the metabolic disorders.

"SUGAR SUGAR ARTERIES CLOG WITH HEAVY LOAD,
ARTERIES BATTLING UNNECESSARY LOAD.
SUGAR SPIKES HATH THE INSULIN LOAD,

*THUS AWAITING THE DIABETIC LOAD.
SWEET SWEET SUGAR CAUSES THE WAISTLINE LOAD"*

BY DR. MAYA MODI

Eat less Sugar You are Sweet Already

Sugar a cause for the insulin resistance in our body and thus hitting the pancreas to outpour more insulin and oh the diabetes is in your basket.

Sugar Spikes Affect the Body

Sugar clogs the arteries and the heart pumps less blood causing the following effects

a] Stenosis of Valves

b] Arrhythmias

c] Cardiac Arrest

d] Diabetes

e] Weight Gain

f] Hypertension

g] Fatty Liver Disease

h] Stroke

i] Increase in Bad Cholesterol LDL

j] Sugar is bad as it is full of calories and has negative effect on brain. The brain uses more energy than any other part in the body and its primary source of energy is glucose.

Effects of sugar on brain

a] The cognitive function is reduced.

b] One's memory is diminished.

c] There are defects in attention seeking factor.

d] It affects self control and emotion.

e] It causes inflammation of brain.

This inflammatory damage to the brain can be reversed by low sugar intake and low glycemic foods.

So the foods with high glycemic index causes elevation in blood glucose. This produces a greater addictive drive in the brain. Thus this causes greater brain activity in regions invoked in, eating behavior, rewards and cravings.

It is said that sugar is much worse than any other product. These days so many come out with ready foods

Sugar Addiction

A] It has been seen that overtime greater amounts of the substance are required to reach the same level of reward.

B] A study implies that over eating results in a diminished response and a progressively worsening addiction to low nutrient foods rich in sugar, salt and fats.

C] A study shows that sweet foods can be more addictive than "cocaine" and was shown in a research in animals.

D] Diabetes and sugar addiction: In a study it was found that Type2 Diabetic people reported with "increased feeling" of sadness and anxiety during acute hyperglycemia [elevated blood sugar] attack.

E] The clogging of blood vessels is the major cause of the vascular complication in diabetics.

F] What happens when you stop eating sugar: When you stop having sugar for a month there are withdrawal symptoms for the first few days. You may have headache feel achy and tired. After the first week you will start feeling better and subsequently you will notice increased energy levels.

G] There is retinopathy of the eyes.

H] The clogging of the arteries causes' loss of sensation in the nerves leads to neuropathy. HbA1c levels have been associated with a greater degree of brain shrinkage.

I] High sugar levels reduce the production of Brain-Derived Neurotrophic Factor [BDNF].

This is a brain chemical more essential for new memory formation and learning. Low levels of BDNF are linked to Dementia, Alzheimer's disease.

J] Sugar and Skin - there is breakdown of collagen and elastin in your skin which is not reversible. There is also Acne, rosacea and eczema of the skin. [they are pimples, skin eruptions and infection of the skin]

Summary for Sugar

A] One must have less sugar.

B] Don't go for added sugars. All readymade foods consist of added sugars.

C] Take fruits as it contains less sugar.

D] Honey and maple syrup can be used in small amounts and are more nutrient.

E] Do not cut off sugar totally.

The US Dietary guideline says that an adult man eating 2000 calories per day will require 50gms of added sugar.

Women should have less sugar up to 30gms / day.

Remember to take jaggery or honey in tea, which is much better.

I now love the use of jaggery in tea and have limited my sugar intake.

B] Hypertension / Blood Pressure

Hypertension kills so many people because it contributes to death from a variety of causes like heart attack, kidney failure, stroke and diabetes.

Blood pressure is measured as 110/70 mm of hg. 110 is the systolic blood pressure. It is the pressure in your arteries as your blood pumps from the heart. 70 is the diastolic blood pressure. It is the pressure in your arteries while the heart is resting between two beats.

The American Heart Association defines normal systolic pressure under 120 and diastolic pressure under 80 or 120/ 80 mm of hg. Values above 140/90 are Hypertensive. Values in between are considered as Pre Hypertensive.

Hypertension puts a strain on the blood vessels and affects the heart. Hypertension causes damage to the eyes, the brain and the kidney. At times it leads to ballooning of the artery [called as aneurysm] and rupture of it. This happens to be the number one killer disease.

The Culprit Causing Hypertension
Soft drinks and empty calories fail health and promote death. But soda is not as deadly as ham bacon sausages and hamburgers. Processed meat is blamed for the deaths of hundred thousand people every year. This figure is four times more people dying world wide than dying from drugs.

Foods for Hypertensives

Eat more Grains:	Saves 1.7 million lives / year.
Eat more Vegetables:	Saves 1.8 million lives / year.
Eat more Nut and Seeds:	Saves 2.5 million lives / year.
Eat more Fruits:	Saves 4.9 million lives / year.

A research has shown low sodium diet, around whole plant foods-whole grains, beans, fruits, dark leafy vegetables and other greens could maintain their blood pressure in normal range even after crossing 60 years of age. Vegetables and other natural foods provide a small amount of sodium you need in your diet.

So High Blood Pressure appears to be a choice.

Salt is the Culprit

This was good until salt was used as a preservative and thus there are added salts to the foods.

Summary for Hypertension

One must take less salt on daily basis and eat healthy foods.

Avoid Stress
And
Exercise Regularly

C] Heart Health - Cardio Vascular Diseases

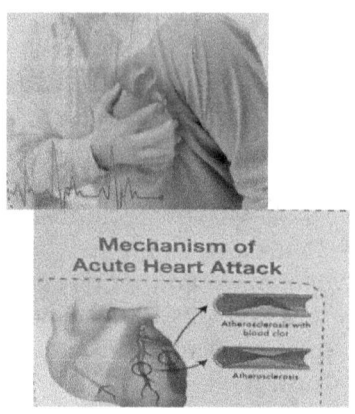

Signs and Symptoms of Chest Pain

Pain Or Discomfort In Chest	Light Headiness	Nausea Or Vomiting	Jaw Neck Or Back Pain
Shortness Of Breath	Cold Clammy Skin	Discomfort Or Pain In Arm Or Shoulder	Just feeling of unwell

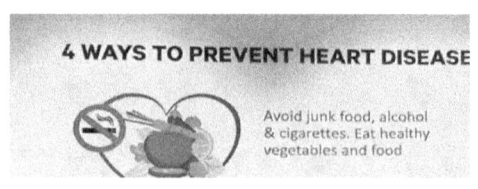

Exercise well.

Do daily yoga.

Sleep well to remain stress free. Mind your mind and your heart will be fine

Don't miss your daily medicine.

Foods to avoid for Heart Disease

Bacon Sausages, Processed Meats	Ice Cream, Pastries, desserts	Fast Food, snacks	Fried Foods
Too Much Salt	All Energy Drinks	Too Much Protein	

Heart disease accounts for nearly one-third of all deaths worldwide. Diet plays a major role in heart health and can impact your risk of heart disease.

Foods to Maximize your Heart Health

Spinach	Kale	Collard greens	Leafy greens reduces risk of disease by 16%
Whole Grains	Whole Wheat	Brown Rice, oats, rye	Read Labels for Whole Grain or Whole Wheat Indicate A Whole Grain Product
Barley	Buck Wheat	Quinoa	3 More Servings of Whole Grains Lowers Risk of Disease By 22%

Words like "wheat flour" or "multigrain" may not really contain whole grain

Heart healthy foods:

Strawberries, blueberries, raspberries	Berries reduce oxidative stress. and	Garlic Has a Compound Called Allicin Which Has Multitude of Therapeutic Effects

	bad cholestrol		
Avocados are an excellent source of heart healthy monounsaturated fats.	Fatty fish, fish oil. Eating salmon 3 times a week reduced diastolic blood pressure significantly	Fish oil reduces blood triglycerides, improves arterial function, decrease blood pressure	Walnuts, rich fiber source, magnesium, copper, manganese
Beans contain resistant starch which decreases levels of cholesterol, triglycerides	Tomatoes Are Loaded With Lycopene, Which Prevents Free Radicals, and Reduces Oxidative Stress	Almonds: Eating 43gm Of Almonds For Six Weeks Reduces Bad Cholesterol.	Chia Seeds, Flex Seeds, Hemp Seeds Are Heart Healthy Having Fiber, Omega3.
Edamame, olive oil	Green Tea, Dark Chocolate	Keep Weight In Check Or Reduce Obesity	Regular Exercise

Summary for Heart Disease

There is definitely a link between diet and heart disease.

What you put on your plate can influence just about every aspect of heart health, from blood pressure and inflammation to cholesterol levels and triglycerides.

Do not let your heart slip. Mind your mind and your heart will be fine. If you don't mind your mind and fill the mind with hatred, jealousy, hatred, ego, depression etc, you will die of heart attack very soon. The cause of heart attack is not block but a bad mind. It is the bad mind that attracts a clot and the clot kills.

Learn to mind your mind.

D] OBESITY: Obesity Kills

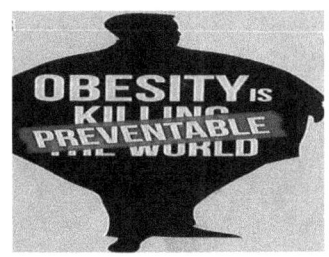

Obesity

The world is getting fatter. There were 250 million people obese in 1980 and now 250 million people in 2019.

How do you know whether you are overweight?

Calculate your body mass index [BMI].

Using this formula BMI = Weight in Kgs / Height in Mtrs.

Score For

Underweight BMI = < 18.5.

Normal BMI	=	18.5 to 24.9
Overweight BMI	=	25 to 29.9
Obesity BMI	=	> 30
Severe obesity BMI	=	> 35

Simple Rules to Stay in Shape: Adopt new Healthy Habits

Good Habits	Bad Habits
Walk, Take a Bike to Work, Balanced Diet, Swim	Drive to Work, Fast Food, Watch T.V Most Of The Time
Balance Your Calorie with Physical Activity	Drinking Beverages full of calories
Control Your Weight Gain	Putting On Weight, over Eating
Dance, Take the Stairs, Do Daily Chores	Watching Movies, On the Laptop or Mobile All The Time

Complications of Obesity

Coronary Heart Disease	Stroke, pulmonary disease	Cataracts	Cancer
Gall Bladder Disease	Non Alcoholic Fatty Liver Disease	indigestion	Inability to Walk
Type 2 Diabetes	Decreased fertility, sexual problems	Osteoarthritis, weak bones	Sleep Apnea

Treating Obesity

The first and foremost is dietary changes

First Is How Many Calories You Take	Make a Chart as to Where You Can Cut Your Calorie Intake	1200 To 1500 Calories for Women	1500 To 1800 Calories for Men, Large Portion Of Food With Fewer Calories
Cut Down On Your Intake of Salt. No alcohol	Eat more Fruits Vegetables, high fibre foods and Coconut	Take Lean Proteins As Beans, Lentil, Soy	Lean Meats are good. If You Like Fish, then Take It Twice a Week
Avoid High Glycemic Foods	Avoid Fats, Dense Carbohydrates, take small amounts of fat from heart healthy fats	Meal Replacement Low Calorie Shake, Healthy Snacks, A Healthy Third Meal That's Low in Fat, Calories	Limit Beverages, Totally Avoid Cakes, Pastries, Fast Food, Fried, Burger, Sausages, Ready To Eat Foods
Be Wary Of Fad Diets. They Do Not Work, There Is Rebound with Increase In Weight	Aim for Short Goals, But For Life Long For Significant Weight Loss, 300 Minutes or More Workout Per Week	Increase Physical Activity, Exercise Is Essential To Reduce Weight	150 Minutes A Week Of Moderate-Intensity Physical Activity To Maintain Weight
Obesity: Any Extra Movement Is Also Efficient Way to	Find Out Factors for the Cause of Obesity, Treat the Cause	Counseling, Support Group Are Essential	Prescription weight Loss Medication Can Be Taken from Your Doctor

Burn Calories			

Bariatic surgery in severe cases of obesity; ballooning and banding of stomach are also done

Summary

Obesity is a killer disease. At time there may be a functional disease too. At such times do take the help of a doctor. Other treatments include banding operation which is also useful.

Chapter 13

Foods to Maintain your Iron

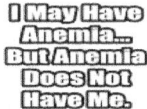
I May Have Anemia... But Anemia Does Not Have Me.

Iron deficiency is the most common and wide spread nutritional disorder in the world, and in India, it affect more than 600 million people. India has high prevalence of iron deficiency anemia is largely due to the local vegetarian diet. Deficiency of iron causes anemia. It is an essential mineral and forms our hemoglobin.

Our body needs Iron to make other hormones too.

Iron is made up of two types
a] Haem Iron
b] Non-Haem Iron.

The Haem Iron is readily absorbed. The Non-Haem Iron is present in vegetables and cannot be absorbed very well. We all know iron plays a vital role in our body iron is required in making hemoglobin and which in turn carries oxygen to all the parts of the body.

Deficiency of Iron

Anemia Decreased Hemoglobin	Soreness, Swelling Of the Mouth	Headaches, Dizziness, paleness,	Heavy Cyclic Bleeding In Females

Levels		Excessive Sweating	
Breathlessness	Increased Heart Rate	Blood Loss Due To Worm Infestations	Damaged Skin
Tiredness	Brittle, Dry Hair	Spoon Shaped Nails [Koilonychias]	Decreased Immunity

Hemolysis of Blood Due To Malarial Infection	Restlessness in Legs	Cold hands and feet	Irrational behavior

There are strange cravings with Iron deficiency like eating ice, clay, dirt, chalk or paper.

Foods with Iron

Legumes, beans, lentils, whole grains	Spinach is a Super Food with Good Amount of Iron	Banana, peaches, apples, oranges pomegranate	Dark Leafy Vegetables .pumpkin,
Green Collards	Kale	Dried Apricots	Tofu
Soy Beans	Hemp	Yogurt	Oats
Cornflakes		Mulberries	Figs
Pear	Prunes	Raisins	Pistachios
Black Currants	Dates	Eggs	Low Fat Milk
Sesame Seed	Pumpkin Seeds	Olives	Peanut Butter
Onions	Dark Chocolate	Coconut Milk	Dried Thyme
Oysters	Chicken Boiled	Mushrooms	Turkey

	Or Roasted		
Cauliflower Green Leaves Carrot Leaves Contain A Good Amount Of Iron	Wheat, bajra, jowar, maize, ragi	**Fruits Contain Less Amount of Iron**	Liver Fried or Roast Kidney
Cheddar Cheese Buffalo Milk Contain Same Amount of Iron	**Cow Milk, Cottage Cheese Have less Amount Of Iron**	**Almonds, Brazil Nuts, Cashews, Coconut Flesh Same but Lesser Amount of Iron**	**Artichokes, Brussel Sprouts, Cabbage, Carrot Raw Little Less of Iron**

Iron Absorption

To increase the Iron absorption of the foods above one must take Vit-C rich foods with it. Sour lemon squeezed on food is an inexpensive and palatable form of taking Vit-C which promotes Iron absorption.

Prevention

Besides food, to increase hemoglobin the iron supplements with zinc are needed. It is very essential to take a deworming tablet prior to treatment of anemia. Parasites are associated with iron-deficiency anemia and they are Hookworms, whipworms and schistosomes. Each Ankylostoma duodenale worm may cause a daily blood loss of 0.2ml which is 10 times more than that caused by Nectar americanus another worm. Heavy hookworm infestation causes blood loss up to 250ml which is equivalent to a daily loss of 29mg of iron.

Severe infestations with whipworms cause blood loss up to 8.5ml.

Supplement of 10mg Iron daily prevents iron-deficiency anemia. Most authorities agree that more expensive iron preparations and quick- or slow-release have no advantage over ferrous sulphate preparations. Ferrous sulphate [100mg tablets] is inexpensive, yet effectively prevents anemia.

Food items for a patient with Anemia

Bread or chapattis or wheat, rice, maize, jowar [sorghum millet] bajra [pearl millet] or ragi [finger millet]

Breakfast cereals of wheat, rice, oatmeal or maize, salads and cooked vegetables, cooked rice, lentils, pulses or beans
Potato, sweet potato and yam and spinach are good
Meat, fish, chicken especially liver kidney and bone marrow

Soup especially liver soup - Eggs, milk and milk products

Fat for cooking and butter - Sugar jaggery or honey.

Sugar intake in moderation - Fruits, fresh fruits, dried especially raisins, currants, dried figs and prunes.

Fruits, fresh fruits, fruits dry especially raisins, currants, dried figs pomegranate, citric fruits, prunes and nuts. Take juices and fluids liberally.

Foods to take in moderation

The sweets, pastries, cakes, cold drinks and desserts are to be taken once in a while. Condiments and spices are to be taken in moderation. Papad chutney or pickle in moderation.

Sample Menu for a Patient with Anemia

Courtesy Clinical Dietetics and Nutrition Philip Abrahim @ F.P. Anita]

Western Diet	Vegetarian Diet	
Breakfast		
Orange Juice	Orange Juice	
Fortified Cereal With Milk	Stewed Prunes	
Scrambled Egg	Fortified Cereal With Milk	
Toast With Jam	Toast Butter Or Wheat Tortilla/Ghee	
Tea Or Coffee	Tea Or Coffee	
Mid-Morning		
Tea Or Coffee	Tea Or Coffee	
Biscuits	Nuts	
Lunch		
Corned Beef Sandwich	Vegetable Cutlets	
Salad: Lettuce, Cucumber, Or Tomato	Wheat Bread Of Coarse Flour	
Spinach	Rice And Curry Of Lentils	
Ice Cream	Milk Pudding	

Mid-Afternoon	
Tea Or Coffee	Tea Or Coffee
Almond Cake	Walnut Cake

Dinner	
Braised Lamb's Liver	Lentil Soup
Minted Potatoes	Beans Risotto
Sliced Green Beans	Salad: Tomatoes, Cucumber, Lettuce, Carrots
Fruit Salad, Yogurt	Vegetable, Purees

Summary

Iron supplements are very essential for treating anemia otherwise it leads to many other complications in health.

With foods other supplements with zinc, folic acid and Vit-B is required.

The doctor decides the length of the treatment and your blood profile would tell as to what has to done.

Chapter 14

Foods for Muscle Cramps

Cramps, Muscle Pain, Spasm

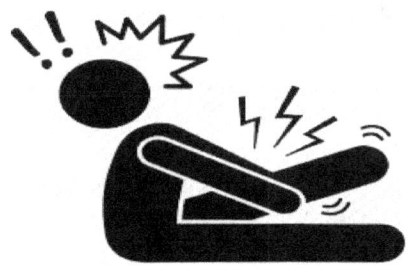

Muscle cramps are painful, clutching and very devastating. There is an electrolyte imbalance of sodium, potassium, chloride, calcium and magnesium.

Causes of Muscle Cramps

Dehydration, Lack of Magnesium	Loss of Electrolytes	Diarrhoea	Lack of stretching Prolonged physical activity
Accumulation of acid	Narrowing of spinal cord	Nerve damage	Diabetic neuropathy

Signs and Symptoms
Sharp pain and severe tenderness in the calf muscles, claudication of muscle due to blockage

of arteries, pain on walking [neurogenic claudication], and heel pain can cause calf muscle tenderness.

Management of Cramps

When having cramps you must drink plenty of water. Hydrate yourself well. Drinking electoral powder is helpful as it helps to balance the electrolytes.

Coconut Water

Coconut water is full of potassium, sodium, magnesium and phosphorus.

Avocado:

Avocado has potassium and magnesium which plays a role in muscle health including muscle contraction.

Water Melon

Water melon contains 92% water and sugars so an excellent choice to hydrate oneself.

Sweet Potato

Sweet potatoes are packed with potassium, calcium and magnesium that are vital for muscle function. 1 cup [200mg] of mashed sweet potato = 20% of the recommended intake of potassium and 13% of recommended intake for magnesium.

Greek Yogurt

Yogurt contains potassium, phosphorous, protein and calcium which is needed for muscle function and the protein helps in muscle repair.

Bone Broth

Broth with apple cider vinegar is a good hydrant and also prevents muscle cramping. It is full of calcium, magnesium and sodium.

Papaya
Papayas are high in magnesium and potassium. 11 ounces [310] gms papaya = 19% @ 15 % magnesium and potassium.

Beet Greens
Beet green is rich in potassium, magnesium, calcium, phosphorus and B vitamins. 1 cup of beet greens = 20% of recommended potassium and magnesium.

Fermented Foods
The fermented foods are pickles, khimchi, and sauerkraut is rich in sodium which helps prevent muscle cramps.

Salmon and Sardines
They are rich in calcium, iron, potassium, magnesium, sodium, phosphorus, and selenium which will improve strength and function of the muscles.

Smoothies
Smoothies can be customized according to needs and taste. Frozen berries + spinach + Greek yogurt + almond butter are supposed to be very nutritive.

Important for Calf Pain
When you have calf pain then try to massage with pain oils or ointments from ankle upward to the calf muscle. Try to keep the leg a bit high so there is reverse flow of blood. A research has

shown that when you have the right side of calf muscle cramps, you should lift your left hand up above the head in lying down position. When you have left side of calf muscle cramps you should lift your right hand above head in lying position.

Summary for Muscle Cramps
Hydrate yourself with plenty of fluids, slow down on exercises, have the above mentioned fruits, coconut water. Magnesium is important, so eat papaya, banana etc.
Spinach is like a miracle veggie.
Potassium will help a lot to relieve cramps.

Chapter 15

Foods for Fatigue

Pep Up Your Energy

Fatigue is feeling of over tiredness or low in energy. There is a strong desire to sleep and this interferes with the normal activity. There is a drain in physical and mental energy. The causes of fatigue are many. Do not let it catch you.

Causes of Fatigue

Over Burdened With Daily Chores	Multi Tasking	Working Women, Home Makers	Physical Exertion beyond Limits, arthritis
Stress, Grief anxiety,	Lack of sleep	Depression	Boredom, obesity
Low Intake of Sugar or Low Intake Of Salt	Hypothyroidism	Alcohol Use	Consumption of Too Many Refined Carbohydrates
Bleeding Disorders	Poor Nutrition	Anemia	Myalgia, Pain in the Muscle
Flu, Cold	Auto Immune Disease	Cancer	Diabetes

In all this we will be treating the causative factor.

Signs and Symptoms of Fatigue

| No Energy, dizziness | Always Feeling Tired | No Inclination to Do Anything | Feeling Sleepy, |

			irritability
No Motivation, moodiness	Weakness of Muscles	Slow Reflexes And Responses	Impaired Decision Making

Food Fix Fatigue

First and foremost I would say nothing is available then just take a small tea spoon of salt with water, it gives good results. Lie down on your bed and keep your head low, below the pillow. This allows more blood flow to the head.

Sugars

Try and take simple fructose as it is better and quickly absorbed and gives instant energy. Now the game plan is to take tea or coffee with sugar.

The advantage of it is that caffeine stimulates the central nervous system which in turn orders the supra renal glands to secrete adrenaline. This in turn will give you more energy.

This in turn also causes the heart to beat faster and thus more oxygenation to the stressed different tissues of the body.

The cell has a component called mitochondria responsible for combining glucose [sugar in the blood] with oxygen thus producing energy, water and carbon dioxide.

This is beneficial as the liver will discharge its glucose into the blood stream in moments of emergency.

Other Foods for Fatigue

| Banana, apple | Lime, ice | Eggs, Jal jeera | Reduce |

	cream		stress
Grains Will Give You Slow Release of Energy	Lean Protein, fish	Protein Powder These Will Energize You the Next Day,	Chicken, Turkey
Bonito Broth Are Good Energizers	Plenty of Water	Complex Carbohydrates	Good Sleep,

Along with foods it is necessary to do life style changes. One should become active, can walk, do different chores, or spot jogging, no fasting, and eat enough calories, frequent meals, proteins to boost your metabolism, positive thinking and multivitamins.

Take Ginseng, chromium with calcium, minerals, Vit-D3 and amino acids. Talk to your doctor.

Summary for Fatigue

One must eat dense carbohydrates with proteins.

De-stress yourself and have adequate sleep.

Take a multivitamin tablet.

Also one should end up having frequent meals.

Chapter 16

Food for Nails

The Showy Healthy Nails

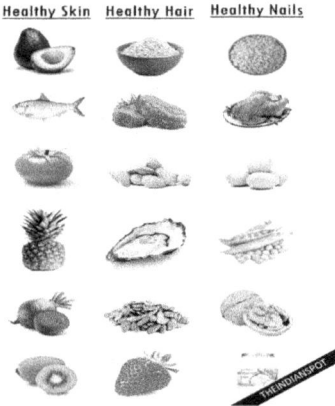

The structure of your nail relies on your nutrition, general health and genetics.

The nutrients can change the nails from dry and brittle to shiny and smooth.

Lack of Moisture
Many have pronounced ridge on the nails. They may have white spots of a powdery finish. They are dry nails. Just rejuvenate them.

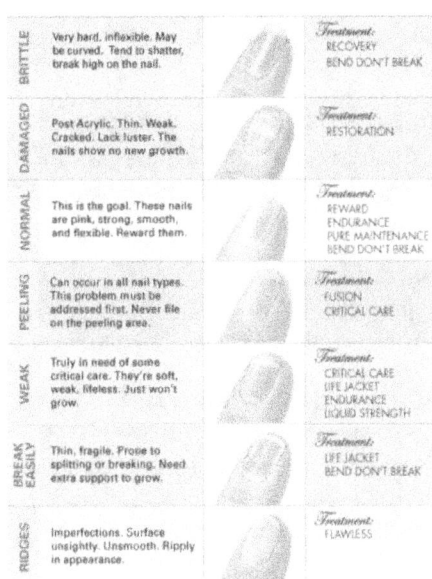

BRITTLE	Very hard, inflexible. May be curved. Tend to shatter, break high on the nail.	*Treatment:* RECOVERY BEND DON'T BREAK
DAMAGED	Post Acrylic. Thin. Weak. Cracked. Lack luster. The nails show no new growth.	*Treatment:* RESTORATION
NORMAL	This is the goal. These nails are pink, strong, smooth, and flexible. Reward them.	*Treatment:* REWARD ENDURANCE PURE MAINTENANCE BEND DON'T BREAK
PEELING	Can occur in all nail types. This problem must be addressed first. Never file on the peeling area.	*Treatment:* FUSION CRITICAL CARE
WEAK	Truly in need of some critical care. They're soft, weak, lifeless. Just won't grow.	*Treatment:* CRITICAL CARE LIFE JACKET ENDURANCE LIQUID STRENGTH
BREAK EASILY	Thin, fragile. Prone to splitting or breaking. Need extra support to grow.	*Treatment:* LIFE JACKET BEND DON'T BREAK
RIDGES	Imperfections. Surface unsightly. Unsmooth. Ripply in appearance.	*Treatment:* FLAWLESS

Jessica Nail Analyst Chart

Foods to Enhance the Nails

Milk Has Vit-D, Calcium and Protein	Banana Has Biotin that Strengthens Brittle Nails	
Biotin Is Present In Organ Meats, salmon, egg yolk	Cauliflower Keeps the Skin around Your Nails Healthy	
Black Discoloration of Nails is Corrected By eating Eggs; this is due To Vit-B12 Deficiency. So take Two Eggs Everyday For One Month will cure it.	Avocado, sweet potato, Palak	**Nuts, Seeds**

Iron is needed to provide your cells with adequate oxygen which is necessary for healthy nails. Iron is obtained from beef, chicken, fish, eggs, dark leafy vegetables, peanuts, beans, spinach.

Important for Nails
Eating oranges or strawberries along with spinach salad with beans and seeds improves iron absorption.

Magnesium for Nails
The vertical ridges on your nails are a sign of magnesium deficiency.

Take Supplement of Magnesium
Dosage 400-420 mg / day for men
Dosage 310-320 mg / day for women.

Magnesium Foods for Nails

Banana	Whole Grains Especially Whole Wheat	Dark Green Leafy Veggies
Peanuts	Edamame, quinoa, almonds	Black Beans

It cures ridges and help formation of new nails.

Protein for Nails
Adequate intake of protein is required to produce Keratin. This is responsible for keeping your nails strong and resilient.

Proteins are obtained from

Meat	Poultry, eggs	Fish	Beans
Lentils Soy	Legumes	Protein Powder	Protein Biscuits

Omega-3 fatty acids for Nails

Omega-3 helps lubricate your nails and gives shiny appearance.

The RDA recommendation for Omega-3 is - 1.6 Gms/ day for men and 1.1 gms / day for women.

Foods with Omega3 for Nails

Tuna	Salmon	Trout	Sardines	
Walnuts	Soy	Eggs	Chia Seeds	Flax Seed and Flax Seed Oil

Vit-C for Nails

It is essential for collagen production, which helps provide strength and integrity to our nails.

Vit-C foods for Nails

All Citrus Fruits	Bell Peppers [Has Good Amount of Vit-C]	Tomatoes, Kiwi	Lemons, Amla, pickles
Fish	Poultry	Eggs	Chick Peas, Black Beans

Summary for Nails

Nutritive foods are important.

Bell peppers are a great source of Vit-C. Cauliflower, spinach are really wonder foods.

Your nails will tell your true tale.

Chapter 17

Foods For Under Eyes- The Dark Circles

The eyes are the most expressive and beautiful part of your face.
Eyes can speak volumes.

The creams and serums don't show their magic unless your pep yourself with nutrients.

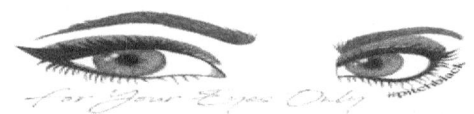

Some Under Eye Packs
Tomatoes can be put under the eyes to lighten the color of the skin. It contains lycopene, lutein, quercetin and beta-carotene.

Tomato juice with a squeeze of lemon is good for the under eyes. Green tea bags as a pack for the eyes.

Cucumber for Eyes
Cucumber hydrates the eyes. Refrigerate the cucumber and apply on eyes which shall give a cool and chilling effect.

Similarly water melon juice or even papaya is good.

Foods for Eyes
Eat tomatoes and lemons daily in food.

Cucumber for Eyes
Try and eat cucumber daily. It is rich in silica, sulphur, vit-A, C, E, and K. This is a classic food. It hydrates the eyes, silica is collagen boosting and sulphur strengthens the skin. It has a coolant effect on eyes and reduces the puffiness.

Guava for Eyes
Guava has Vit-C and antioxidants. Avocados has Vit-E and healthy fats so prevents dryness around the eyes.

Mulberry for Eyes
It has resveratrol which is an age defying antioxidant. It is rich in Vit-A, B1, B2 and Vit-C, iron and copper. This is excellent and helps lighten the skin under the eyes.

Blueberries for Eyes
The Vit-C, antioxidant and omega-3 fatty acids of the berries help regulate and increase the blood circulation near the eyes and protect the vessels. The manganese helps the lightening of the skin.

Goji berries for Eyes
They are loaded with lots of nutrients Vit-B, Vit-C, beta carotene, iron, copper, zeaxanthin, polysaccharides and minerals. They too protect the blood vessels and boost the skin around the eyes. Key nutrients are lycopene, potassium and magnesium.

Watermelon for Eyes

It is rich in water, Vit-B, B6, Vit-C, antioxidants and beta-carotene. This acts as a hydrant to the eyes.

Celery for Eyes
It is rich in sodium, potassium, magnesium quercetin and fiber. This is a powerful fluid regulator and can help reduce Puffiness. The sodium in celery is different than table salt. The sodium helps in absorption of the nutrients.

Beetroot for Eyes
It has folate too with Vit-C, magnesium and betalain pigment. So these are good for the eyes.

B A O B A B for Eyes
This is a fruit with impressive health benefits. The baobab fruit and the powder are widely recognized as SUPERFOOD. It is a rich source of omega-3 fatty acid and is a good choice for the sensitive and inflamed skin. It has low sodium levels, balances fluids and prevents puffiness of eyes.

Bee pollen for Eyes
They are rich in 18 vitamins all of which are Amino acids, fatty acids and proteins. It is sold in granules. Take 1tsf of it daily. One can add it to yogurt or smoothie, but it tastes a little bitter. It is beneficial to the eyes and for overall health.

Caution
It is not to be given to children, pregnant women, breast feeding mother and person who has bee sting allergy.

Spirulina for Eyes

It is full of proteins, antioxidants, fatty acids, B vitamins, calcium and sulphur.

The protein helps in the renewal of the tissue. Sulphur is known to strengthen the skin. Dose ¼ tsf daily and increase it to 1tsf daily.

> Tablet Centrum and Vigorex works wonderfully for the eyes.

Summary for Eyes

Apart from these nutrients one needs to relax and My personal experience is use of tablet Centrum or cap vigorex.

In preventing dark circles and also helps in delaying wrinkles setting in on the face and crow's feet. It gives amazing results.

Also get enough sleep. No smoking. Learn to destress yourself well.

Hydrate oneself with water and reduce salt intake.

Believe in your heart that you are meant to live a life full of passion, purpose, magic and miracles.

The purpose of life is to be happy and healthy.

The purpose is to be useful, to be honorable, to have it and make some difference that you have lived and lived well.

Part 3

Chapter 18

Sleep -Night Armor

Sleep Better and Smarter

We already talked about, why the food is important and what you need to do it and besides them other things accompanying are essential as well.

Sleep Smarter and Better
Sleep time is the most essential factor. Many of us sacrifice our sleep time to get more work done but in doing so you are disturbing the fundas of good health.

It is a proven fact that lack of sleep or less sleep impacts ones decision making and not only that it even makes wayward decision regarding your food.

Sleep is the missing factor for weight gain shown in a study in United States.

Mechanism of Eating at Night
The two hormones that help regulate hunger grehlin and leptin are affected by sleep. Grehlin

stimulates appetite while leptin reduces it. So grehlin signals your body for more food. When you sleep less, your body makes more grehlin, and it signals the brain to eat more. Leptin is a hormone for fullness. But when there is lack of sleep there is more grehlin and the leptin levels are further lowered, thus one ends up eating more. So you mess yourself up by eating foods.

A study in American Journal of Nutrition quoted that lack of sleep caused one to eat high carbohydrate or high fat foods. Too little sleep lowers your metabolism and decreases the insulin sensitivity, thus the body is unable to metabolize your fats and carbohydrate. So again more weight gain. So a sleep deprived brain will make you snack more at night.

Sleep Better

A person needs 7 to 9 hours of sleep regularly. Getting sleep less than this is detrimental to health. The brain fog that occurs due to that make you eat.
One needs to understand the sleep cycle properly.

There are two types of sleep
1] Non Rapid Eye Movement [NREM]
2] Rapid Eye Movement [REM].

NREM sleep is divided into 1, 2, 3 and 4 stages. A complete sleep cycle takes an average of 90 minutes. The second and latter cycles are long lasting approximately 90-120 minutes. [Carskadon and Dement, 2005].

Stage 1 Sleep

This stage of sleep is light with rolling of eyes and can be disturbed easily to drift out of sleep. It is a wakeful relaxation stage may be precedent by muscle contraction. If you awaken someone during this stage, they might report that they were not really asleep.

Stage 2 Sleep

It lasts approximately 10 to 25 minutes in the initial cycle and lengthens with each successive cycle. Here the rapid eye movement is stopped and the body prepares for deep sleep. There is also slowing of heart rate and a little fall of body temperature. You become less aware of your surroundings. The brain spindles become slower with occasional burst of rapid brain waves.

Stage 3 Sleep

This is referred to as slow wave sleep. It is characterized by slow wave activity called delta waves. The muscles relax, blood pressure drops and breathing rate also slows down. Now is the time of deepest sleep. The person can do night walking, experience terror, talk in sleep and bed wetting. Here people become less responsive to noises and activity and may fail to generate a response.

Stage 4 Sleep

The arousal stage is highest in this stage. Awakening as this time will lead to disorientation.

REM SLEEP

Dreaming is often associated with REM sleep. Loss of muscle tone and reflexes serves as an important function because it prevents an individual from acting out their dreams or nightmares while sleeping. Approximately 80% of vivid dream recall results after arousal from this stage of sleep [dement and kleitman1957] the brain becomes more active. The body becomes relaxed and immobilized. The eyes move rapidly.

REM SLEEP
It is characterized by eye movement, increased respiration rate and increased brain activity and muscles become more relaxed.

The stages 3 and 4 are important for good sleep. Hence if you sleep adequately in the afternoon your night sleep is disturbed. We must learn to sleep in complete cycles and the body needs consistency.

How to Sleep Well
All is well when sleep is well.

1] Proper Bed Time
It is essential to sleep in a peaceful environment without any disturbance of external noises.

2] Proper Wake Time
It is essential to sleep at the same time and accordingly you wake up at the same time.

> EARLY TO BED, EARLY TO RISE,
> MAKES A MAN HEALTHY WEALTHY AND WISE.

In case you sleep late or you have disturbed sleep then too try getting up at the same time.

3] Power Naps

The power naps work wonders for me. After a power nap, I am completely fresh, energetic and ready for work.

4] Alcohol

In fact alcohol has the reverse effect, meaning it will hinder your sleep and make you restless. I have experienced it; do not use it to induce sleep.

Even drinking tea or coffee should be avoided late night as it hinders sleep.

5] Comfortable Environment

When sleeping, one must dim the lights, change into your night suit and brush your teeth. Then get into the comfort of your sheets. Turn off electronic devices. Relax close your eyes and try to sleep.

6] Bedroom and Sex

Always keep the bedroom for sole purpose of sex. Here there should be no other hindrance like TV, clock, laptop. Sexsize to get good sleep.

7] Sleep Inducing Foods at Nights

Spinach	Kale	Arugula	Mustard Greens
Cherry Tarts, cheery juice	Banana	Almonds, walnuts	Milk, yogurt
Cheese	Fatty Fish Salmon, Trout, Tuna, Mackerel Increases Serotonin Levels to Induce Sleep	Chamomile Tea Contains Apigenin That Binds To Receptors, Promotes Sleep	Turkey Has Tryptophan . Little Proteins Helps Induce Sleep

Sweeten Your Herbal Tea With Honey. It Raises Insulin, Allows Tryptophan to Enter Your Brain That Help Induce Sleep	Kiwi Is Full Of Serotonin, Helps Sleep Well	Jasmine Rice Has A High Glycemic Index, Induces Sleep Easily	Calcium, Sleep Inducing Tryptophan

8] The Military Method of Sleep

Relax your entire face including the muscles inside your mouth.

Drop your shoulders to release the tension and let your hands drop to the side of your body.

Exhale relaxing your chest.

Relax your legs, thighs and calves.

Clear your mind for 10 seconds by imagining a relaxing scene.

The moment your sleepy rush to your bed.

9] Try Sleep Gadgets

Passion pattern ear plugs, anti snore gadget, a good pillow, nasal strips breathe right, Casper glow technology, aroma sleep.

EARLY TO BED, EARLY TO RISE MAKES A MAN HEALTHY WEALTHY AND WISE.
THIS IS A PHRASE BY POOR RICHARD ALMANACK.

In these days I wonder if it will be followed. But if you can it is the best gift for sleep.

Smart Supplements

We have already talked above the use of smart supplements.

These are taken besides the foods we eat. It is difficult to plan our entire each day for the nutrients and -+ balance from foods.

The bio-availability in the foods is difficult to measure.

Also the absorption of certain nutrients does not work in the presence of others, for example iron and calcium hamper each other's absorption ability. Thus supplements are needed.

I am a fan and take these supplements religiously.

Take Calcium and Vit-D3 for bone health.

Proteins needed for muscle mass

A multivitamin for strength and healthy muscles, whey protein is needed for energy.

Chapter 19

Supplements

The Need Of The Hour

This will full fill all our requirements of the body to keep it fit and running.

I will mention supplements that are available across the counter and without a prescription.

Supplements

Vitamins	What it does	Where it is found	Daily values
Biotin	Energy storage, helps in	Avocados, cauliflower	30 mcg
	Protein, carbs, and fat metabolism	Eggs, raspberry, liver	
		Pork, beef, whole grains	
Choline	Brain development, signaling to cells, fat transport, metabolism, liver, Function, muscle movement, nerve function, normal metabolism	Beans and peas, nuts, milk, soy foods, salmon, cauliflower, Spinach, broccoli and liver.	550 mg
Folate / folic acid	Prevention of birth defects, protein metabolism, red blood cell formation	Beans, peas, avocados, asparagus, cereals, Pasta, rice, green leafy	400 - 600 mcg Or 5-10

		vegetables, Spinach, oranges and orange juice.	mg /day in pregnancy
Niacin helps in	Helps in lightening of the skin, reduces fine wrinkles, and boost collagen formation	Beans, nuts, poultry, seafood, Whole grains, pork, beef cereals, Pasta and rice	16 mg
Pantothenic acid	Conversion of food into energy, fat metabolism, Hormone production, nervous system function, red blood cell formation.	Beans and peas, broccoli, eggs, milk, mushrooms, poultry, seafood, sweet potato, whole grains, yogurt.	5 mg
Riboflavin	Conversion of food into energy, growth and development, red blood cell formation	Milk, mushrooms, eggs, meat, spinach, poultry, sea food, enriched products, bread, cereals, pasta, rice	1.3 mg
Thiamin Vit-B1	Conversion of food into energy, nervous system function	Nuts, whole grains, sunflower seeds, beans and peas, pork, enriched grain products.	1.2 mg
Vit-A	Vision, growth, development, immune function, reproduction, red	Carrots, cantaloupe, eggs, dairy products,	900 mcg 10,000 25,000

	blood cell formation, skin, bone formation.	fortified cereals, green leafy vegetables, spinach, broccoli, pumpkin, red peppers, sweet potato.	I.U per day is fine
Beta carotene	Beta carotene converts into vit-A, good vision, healthy immune system, healthy skin, mucus membrane	Carrots, sweet potato, spinach, kale, apricots, cantaloupe	25,000 / 200,000 I.U.
Vit-B6	Immune function, nervous system function, protein carbohydrate fat metabolism, red blood cell formation	Chick peas, fruits other than citrus, potatoes, Salmon, tuna	1.7 mg
Vit-B12	Conversion of food into energy, Nervous system function, red cell formation	Dairy products, Eggs, Fortified cereals, Meat, Poultry, Sea food clam, salmon tuna.	2.4 mcg
Vit-C	Here is no area that Vit-c does not work. Antioxidant Collagen and connective tissue formation Immune function, Wound healing	All citrus fruits, kiwi and berries, Lemons, Orange, grapefruit and tomato juices and the fruits, Broccoli, Brussel sprouts, bell peppers tomatoes.	90 mg
VIT-D	Bone Growth	Sunlight, Eggs	600

	Calcium Uptake and Balance, Hormone production, Blood pressure regulation, Immune function, Nervous system function.	Fish oil and cod liver oil, Fish-Mackrel, salmon, herring, trout and tuna. Fortified dairy products, Fortified orange juice, Soy, rice, almonds, pork Fortified cereals, Mushrooms	I.U
Vit-E	Antioxidant, Formation of blood vessels, Immune function, Hair skin	Green vegetables-spinach broccoli, Nuts, seeds Peanuts, peanut butter, Vegetable oils	15 mg
Vit-K	Blood clotting Strong bones	All greens, spinach, Greens, broccoli, kale, turnip, greens, collard greens, Swiss chard and mustard greens.	120 mcg
Calcium	Bone, teeth formation, blood clotting constriction, relaxation of blood vessels, Hormone secretion, Muscle contraction, Nervous system function	Dairy products, Low fat Milk, banana, Tofu, Green vegetables, broccoli, collard greens, canned sea food with bones, Fortified orange juice, cereals	1300 mg

Chloride	Acid base balance, conversion of food into energy, digestion, Fluid balance, Nervous system function	Olives, Ryes, Salt substitutes, Seaweeds-use, kelp, Table salt, sea salt Vegetables-celery, lettuce and tomatoes, Water	2300 mg
Chromium	Insulin function Protein, carbohydrates, fat metabolism	Spices-garlic, basil, Broccoli, Meats, turkey, Whole grains Apples, banana, Grape, orange juice	35 mcg
Copper	Antioxidant, Bone formation Collagen and connective tissue formation, Energy production, Iron metabolism, Nervous system function	Chocolate and cocoa, Lentils, Nuts, seeds, Crustaceans, shell fish Organ meats-liver, whole grains	0.9 mg
Iodine	Growth, Development, Metabolism Reproduction Thyroid hormone function	Breads, cereals, Dairy products, Iodized salt, Potatoes, Seafood, Seaweed, Turkey	150 mcg
Iron	Red blood cell formation Energy production Immune function Growth, development	Beans, Eggs, Nuts, Meat, organ meats [liver] Raisins, prunes, dates Spinach,	18 mg

	Reproduction Wound healing	broccoli, bell peppers Peas, Poultry, Seafood-sardines, shrimp, oysters tuna and haddock, Soy products Whole grains, fortified cereals, Jaggery	
Magnesium	Blood pressure regulation, Blood sugar regulation, Bone formation, Energy production. Hormone production, Immune function, Muscle contraction, Nervous system function, Normal heart rhythm, Protein formation	Avocados, Beans and peas Dairy products, Banana and raisins, Green leafy-spinach, Nuts, pumpkin seeds, Potatoes, Whole grains,	420 mg
Manganese	Carbohydrate protein, cholesterol metabolism, Cartilage, bone formation Wound healing	Beans, Nuts Pineapple, Spinach Sweet potato Whole grains	2.3 mg
Molybdenum	Enzyme production	Beans, peas, Nuts, Whole grains	45 mcg
Phosphorus	Acid base balance Bone formation Energy production, storage Hormone activation	Beans, peas, Dairy products, Meat, Nuts, seeds, Poultry, Seafood, Whole	1250 mg

		grain, Enriched, fortified cereals and breads	
Potassium	Blood pressure regulation Carbohydrate metabolism Fluid balance Growth and development Heart function Muscle contraction Nervous system function Protein formation	Beans, peas, Dairy products, low fat milk, cheese, yogurt, Banana, dry apricots, stewed prunes, Carrot, vegetable juices, Orange, prune, pomegranate, fruits, juices, Tomato, its products, Seafood-clams, salmon, Potatoes, sweet potato, beet, greens, spinach, Coconut water, Banana	4700 mg
Selenium	Antioxidant, Immune function, Reproduction Thyroid function	Eggs, Meat, Nuts- Brazil nuts and seeds, Poultry, Seafood, Whole grains, Enriched pasta, rice	55 mcg
Sodium	Acid base balance, Blood pressure regulation, Fluid balance, Muscle contraction Nervous system function	Cheese, Chicken, Cold cuts, cured meats, Breads, rolls, Egg dishes, omelets, Pizza, Sandwiches, hamburgers, hot	2300 mg

		dogs, Soups	
Zinc	Growth and development Immune function, Nervous system function, Protein formation, Reproduction Taste, smell, Wound healing	Beans, peas, Dairy products Beef, Fortified cereals, Nuts, Poultry, Shellfish, Whole grains	11 mg

Source: U.S Food and Drug [FDA] Administration

Chapter 20

Happiness

But Smart Happiness

We have understood foods, sleep vitamins and minerals. Everyone has to now learn to be smart and be happy.

Mood affects our eating and we develop food disorders. When your mood is low one just grabs at an ice-cream, candy, sweets or chocolates. We just get out of control and let our mood be satisfied with foods and end result is, Oh! Gosh! What you see is those extra pounds on your belly which is definitely unhealthy.

Any form of mood disturbance signals the neurotransmitters which affects foods, moods, appetite, thinking and it may make you eat poorly, laze about, avoid exercise.

If you are stressed more then there is extra release of cortisol. Cortisol is the demon that makes you have more cravings for food and energy. All these extra calories are stored on the belly, the Pot Belly.

Now if you are happy you will have higher amounts of Serotonin, also called as the Happiness Hormone. So you will not unnecessary eat or think of food.

So let's fight the enemy, the Cortisol, and Let's Embrace Happiness, The Serotonin. We have heard and learned how to be happy, there are books, sayings and gurus are there but a few things one should incorporate for happiness.

Happiness Starts With The Talk Of Happiness

We always try to search happiness from outside sources. We are happy when our children, parents or partner is happy. When one is free of daily chores, we are happy. Happiness is a harmonious co-ordination between what the heart wills and the rest of the world. We have dreams, desires and the need to fulfill it. Our dreams and desire needs power.

AN OLD SAYING GOES:

WHEN THERE IS A WILL, THERE IS A WAY.

In Doing Something for Self, Leads to Happiness.

Some Fundas for Happiness

Enjoy the joy of light in the sunlight. The sun looks at us with its ambient yellow rays to much satisfaction similarly reach out and enjoy.

Plan a Trip

It is necessary to let yourself free and enjoy nature to release your tensions. Behold the surroundings and walk through with a smile. Enjoy the fragrance of the flowers.

Shopping

This is definitely a mood up lifter for many. I for one enjoy this very much, but I restrict myself to do only window shopping. You're shopping should not sink a hole in your pocket.

In my childhood, I had enacted a song - *There is a whole in my bucket Dear Liza, Reply is Then Mend it Dear Liza.*
So mend your moods to happiness.

Laughter
Laughter is the best medicine. Laugh a while with self and friends. Remember good things to stimulate your brain. There are many laughter clubs around. Join one of them.

Engage Yourself
One good activity is gardening. The oxygen from the plants shall give you joy as the cells are activated and filled with oxygen.

Have Sex
Sex is one of the best activities for mood uplifts and happiness. The neurotransmitter Dopamine is produced in response to sexual stimulation. Thanks to Dopamine we really do feel the enjoyment. The other reason is the logical part of your brain is shut down. It is not the act of orgasm that gives you satisfaction but the fondling and cuddling does it. Not only does it make you happy, it has a host of health and mood improving habits, and the best of all it is an amazing exercise.

Talk to someone
You must talk to someone, whom you can trust completely. This will lessen the burden on you.

A SAYING

'JOY SHARED IS JOY DOUBLED,
AND SORROW SHARED IS SORROW HALVED'.

It may make you see things in better light and even laugh at yourself. One can scribble things on paper too.

Chanting
I have found that chanting loudly and repeating works wonders for the mind body and soul. It will channelize your thoughts and you forget the other ones. Try this, it is very helpful

Hobbies
Have you ever realized that dancing is one of the best sources of happiness? You are engaging yourself in a new activity and concentrating on steps and remembering it, so your mind is diverted, your body feels light, and mood is also elevated. A good exercise too. I am freak for dancing and my major happiness comes through it. Also walk, listen to music, play harmonium, etc. it is engaging the mind to a new entity.

Happiness Foods

Walnuts	Dark leafy vegetables, Dark chocolate having 65% of real cocoa. This ensures that it is less in sugars.	Grass fed beef	Cold water fish, Salmon, tuna Mackerel, herring,
Chia seeds	Fortified foods with omega3	Eggs	Milk and yogurt
Foods rich in Omega 3 fatty acids	Shell fish. Fish consumes phytoplankton, which consumes microalgae, they accumulate	Tilapia, Edamame	Foods rich in Vit-B9 and B6, Food rich in B12

	omega3 in the tissues		

But remember happiness is from within. You are the only person who can make yourself happy. The all other things are accomplishments.

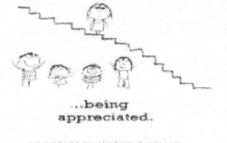

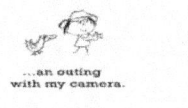

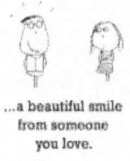

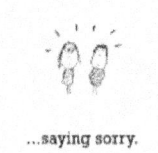

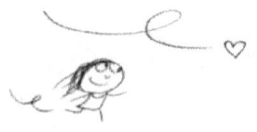

...following
your heart.

Be Happy In All Circumstances

Chapter 21

Exercises - Easy and Smart

Another Breather of Life

Exercise is one of the best forms of investment you can make which would go with you later in life to keep you healthy. It is a long term investment plan.

It depends whether you have been exercising before or not. Is your life style sedentary? Any time, any place, is good to start exercising. Remember to take one step at a time, don't jump into anything.

Start with a simple walk or moving about, do some simple hand lifting exercises. I don't want you to think you are into a weight loss program but a more fitness regime where you will do everything without support. This is the basic idea. Don't target weight.

Start with, simple walking to brisk walking, some stretches, yoga for health, swimming, cycling, running, for those who are able to do it. One can just groove to music by watching on your TV. Dance is a very good form of exercise but depends on one's ability and liking.

1] Walking
Walking is your second heart. Keep walking. The calf muscles in your leg are the second heart.

Everyone knows that the heart pumps blood, right? But did you know that your body has a second blood pump? It's your calf muscles! That's right! The calf muscles in your legs are your second heart!

Walking is good for the heart. A person with heart disease should try walking step by step, increasing the time slowly. In arthritis too walking is beneficial but start when your pain is relieved. It relieves stress and slows down ageing process. It is good for chest infections. Instead of taking a bus walk your way. One must use the staircase instead of lift. Walk ten minutes after meals.

2] Stretching Exercises

Stretching is dynamic and static. Dynamic stretching is done before exercises to make your muscles active. Static stretching is one holds the position for minimum of 10 to 20 seconds. This should be done after exercise to relax the muscles.

Spending time lengthening your limbs also has mental benefits. "Going through a series of stretching can reduce stress and cortisol levels".

GREENFIELD ADDS:
> WHILE THE BEST TIME TO STRETCH IS WHEN MUSCLES ARE WARM-SAY, AFTER A WALK OR A WORKOUT-STRETCHING IS SO BENEFICIAL THAT WHENEVER YOU CAN SQUEEZE IT IN, YOU SHOULD.

3] Hip and knee strengthening exercises:

If you knees are in place, you will be able to walk properly and bear the weight of your body. By working on improving your hip strength and overall balance, you may be able to keep your knees in the correct position and, ultimately, remove your knee pain.

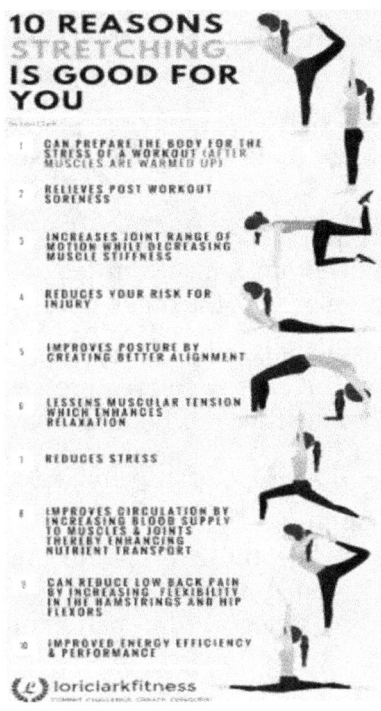

Knee Strengthening Exercises

A] Straight leg raises sleeping or standing position one leg at a time. Your Quadriceps in front of the thigh muscle will get stronger.

B] Hamstring curls the muscles at the back of thighs. Stand in front of a chair, hold it and bend a little forward and curl your leg to touch back of thighs or just short of it. Repeat other side. 10 count each.

C] Wall squats. Wall squats are like sitting in a chair, without the chair but with support of the wall. Can start half sitting also.

D] Step-ups. In your house climb two steps up and come down or just one step up and down.

E] Calf rises. Sleep on the floor with knees bent, open your leg, hold and back, repeat same on other side.

F] Side leg rises. Sleep on the side, with hand under the head and, raise your leg to 45degrees and back similarly on the other side.

G] Leg presses. Sit with legs straight. Now put a 6inch below the knees and then press your knees to it and at same time flex your knees.

Hip Exercises

H] Supine pelvic tilt. Lie on the ground with your legs popped up and body touching the ground. Now squeeze your pelvic muscles up then relax.

I] Bridging. Here lie down knees pulled in legs touching the ground. Now lift your bottom up off the ground just to about level. So you don't want to arch your back and not sagging. Then slowly come back down. You are working your hamstrings, working your gluteus and getting the hips moving.

J] Straight leg rises. Sleep on the ground, one knee in; now slowly lift the other leg just to the level of the other knee.

K] Side crunches for oblique muscles of the abdomen Sleep on the ground with knees in, now put your hand behind the head and raise and turn to the left, then right. Go up with the body.

L] Lying down position with knees in, tighten and push the hip muscles to the right side and then to the left side.

M] Standing side crunches. Stand straight, hands behind the head; raise left leg to touch the right hand while twisting from right to left. Repeat other side.

Upper Body Exercises
This can be done sitting or standing.

1] Namaste: fold your hands in front and press as much as you can.

2] Place both your hands on the back of the buttocks and press your elbow inwards. The trapezes muscle, rhomboid muscle and the scapula are benefitted. This will neck tension from slouching.

3] Hold your hands in prayer position, slowly take it up so that your elbows touch and then bring it down, letting the elbows remain at the same position. The pectorals and biceps and triceps are working

4] Body straight, take your hands out straight and so circular movements clockwise and anticlockwise. Then again hands out and palms facing in front, pump your hands in front and same posture pump them back.

5] Hold a ball and squeeze, this gives strength to wrist and improves the capacity to hold things properly.

6] Along with this hip exercise for strengthening, by doing the bridge exercise, as talked before. Also core strengthening is essential and for that must do side or front plank. You need to learn this.

Importance of Weight Training
Weight training is the best form of exercise for keeping the bones strong and healthy. If you have no weights then there is something like body weight training exercise, resistance band work out, or just use bottles filled with water. This gives strength and builds up your energy.

Another way is climbing of stairs. This can be easily done in the comfort of your home or at the gym.

First learn, train with an instructor. It is necessary that all need to do weight and strength training workouts.

Even women need to build muscles. Weight training is for both men and women.

There are exercise to get a better core like Pilates, yoga, pranayam, abs and core exercises, aerobics, dance, jazz exercises, zumba and endless forms of exercise.

Benefits of Exercise

1] Strengthens muscles,

2] Strengthens lungs,

3] Weight control,

4] Reduced risk of heart disease,

5] Strong immune system,

6] Improved blood pressure,

7] Improved brain function,

8] Better flexibility,

9] Better power, 1

10] Better posture,

11] Better bone density

What Counts As Moderate Physical Activity

1] Walking

2] Gardening

3] Cycling

4] Hiking

5] Dancing

6] Swimming

7] Active recreation

Good to exercise is morning, and if you make it a habit you will not be able to miss it.

Exercise always to your capacity.

Incorporate 20 to 30 minutes of work out four times a week.

First learn the exercises then start it.

Slow and steady wins the race.

Can start with count of 15seconds and rest of 15seconds, and then increase to each exercise for 60seconds.

Slowly increase the set from one to two to three sets of each exercise.

Chapter 22

Meditation is Important

Bring Peace and Calm to Self

Meditation can be defined as a state of technique that are intended to encourage a heightened state of awareness and focused attention. It will really help you change your attitude towards life. And provide peace of mind and happiness. It will help you achieve a better understanding of yourself and others. Since it helps to clear your head, meditation improves your concentration levels, memory creativity and also makes you feel rejuvenated.

Benefits of Meditation
Controls anxiety, promotes emotional health, enhances self awareness, lengthens life span, may reduce age related memory loss, can generate kindness, may help fight addictions, and helps ward off unnecessary stress, no cluttering of people in your mind.

Mindfulness meditation can actually change the structure of the brain. Eight weeks of mindfulness based stress reduction [MSRB] was found to increase cortical thickness in the hippocampus, which governs learning and memory. It can quiet the mind and body while enhancing inner peace. When done before bedtime, meditation may help reduce insomnia and sleep troubles by promoting overall calmness. It decreases blood pressure and abundant holistic benefits.

1] Muldhara Chakra

This is the first Chakra.
Location: Base of the spine.
Basic Issues: Survival, vitality, stability, security.
Color: Red.
Mantra: Lam.
If balanced you feel: Security, humility, grounded, stable, energetic, optimal weight, healthy eating, and proper elimination.
If unbalanced you feel: Insecure, fear, anxiety, unstable, low self esteem, anemia, over/underweight, and constipation.

2] Svadhisthana Chakra

The second chakra which is the the sacral Chakra.
Location: Between genital and pubic bone
Basic issues: Creativity, sexuality, reproduction, pleasure.
Color: Orange.
Mantra: Vam.
If balanced you feel: creativity, joy, sexuality, healthy sex life, prosperity, patience, fertility, and pleasure.
If unbalanced you feel: guilty, shyness, irresponsible, infertility, sexual issues, allergy, and eating disorders.

3] Manipura Chakra

Third chakra - solar plexus Chakra.
Location: Between naval and the breastbone

Basic issues: power, strength, self-esteem, warrior energy.
Color: Yellow.
Mantra: Ram.
If balanced you feel: energy, strength, confidence, strong will, mental balance, health, confidence, active.
If unbalanced you feel: guilty, lack of weakness, allergy, fatigue, low self-esteem, worthlessness, digestion and liver problems

4] Anahata Chakra

The fourth chakra - the heart Chakra.
Location: Centre of the chest.
Basic issues: love, acceptance, compassion.
Color: Green.
If balanced you feel: Loving, empathetic, open-hearted, serenity, emotionally balanced, trustfulness, tolerance.
If unbalanced you feel: loneliness, demanding, critical, jealous, cold hearted, narcissistic, heart and lung problem, asthma, allergies.

5] Vishudhha Chakra

The fifth chakra - the throat Chakra.
Location: Throat
Basic issues: Communication, self expression.
Color: Blue.
Mantra: Hum.
If balanced you feel: Peaceful, powerful, listening, good communication, strong, self expression,
If unbalanced you feel: Shy, weak voice, fear of speaking, unable to listen, lying, arrogance, thyroid, hearing, throat problems.

6] Ajna Chakra

The sixth chakra - third eye Chakra.
Location: Between brows.
Basic issues: Intuition, perception, vision.
Color: Indigo.
Mantra: Om.
If balanced you feel: Intuitive, guided, perceptive, clairvoyance, bright dreams, spiritual, mental strength, good vision,
If unbalanced you feel: Lack of intuition and imagination, manipulative, panic, fear, nightmares, vision and eye problems, migraines.

7] Sahasrara Chakra

The seventh chakra - the crown Chakra.
Location: Top of the head.
Basic issues: Knowing, connection to spirits and universe.
Color: Violet, White.
Mantra: Silence, Om.
If balanced you feel: spiritual, blessed, unity, wisdom, open minded, peaceful, connected to universe, strong nervous system, If unbalanced you feel: mental disorders, fear, materialistic, memory and learning problems, apathy, broken, spiritual crisis.

Types of Meditation

a] Spiritual ,Meditation

b] Mindfulness Meditation

c] Movement Meditation

d] Focused Meditation

e]Visualization Meditation

f] Chanting Meditation

g] Kundalini Meditation

h] Qi Gong Meditation (I am a member of this group.)

i] Vipassana.

There are many more but these are the important ones.

Best Way to Meditate

1] Sit or lie comfortably.
You may even want to invest in a meditation chair.

2] Close your eyes.

3] Make no effort to control the breath, simply breathe naturally.

4] Focus your attention on the breath and on how the body moves with each inhalation and exhalation.

1] Chose a preferable time for meditation especially the night time is good or when you are alone and there is no disturbance. First sit in a comfortable position with dimmed lights. Then close your eyes and focus at the centre of the head. Let yourself flow letting all surrounding sound out of your mind.

2] With your eyes closed start breathing in to pump the air into the abdomen. Breathe for a count of six, hold for a count of six, and then slowly breathe out and take your stomach inside.

3] Now just concentrate on your breathing, inhale and exhale out. Do it three to four times.

4] At times the mind keeps wandering here and there but again can bring it back and concentrate on your breathing. Monitor your breathing. Keep focusing on your breath, it will help to focus.
Make this your daily routine. It empowers you with peace and calm mind.

Solar eclipse meditation. Solar eclipse was not seen in India. It was seen in north and South America from 7.30 to 12.30 am the next day. [Indian time] Solar eclipse is strong, powerful and full of energy. That was the Somvati Amavasya solar eclipse, the name is because solar eclipse was on a Monday. It was the new moon in the south of Sagittarius. The vibes are strong, painful, life changing and preparations were necessary to face them.

First is the Mahadev [Lord Shiva] meditation. To sit in a comfortable position-no distraction-no sound-back straight-shoulders back-hand in mudra style and drop it on your lap-keep chin up-no discomfort-the eyes shut. In systematic manner take a deep breath blowing the stomach and the exhale out taking the stomach in. shut all your thoughts out, observe breath, self talk if you indulge, put an end to it and focus on breathing. Keep breathing in for 6 counts and

Next is chanting of lord Ganesha: Om Ganpati Namah, 5-7 times followed by the Gayatri mantra.

OM BHUR BHUVA SVAH

TAT SAVITUR VARENYAM

BHARGO DEVASYA DHIMAHI

DHIYO YO NAHA PRACHODAYAT

Then there is Surya Namah chant. This is for the sun. Om hrim suryaya Namah mantra. Chant these a few times. Sit in the same way for meditation. Close your eyes and radiate into positive and warm energy of the sun. Imagine the sun with eyes closed. The sun rays on your body and everything is glowing and radiant with energy of sun [Surya]. The surya mantra is mentioned in ancient history. It destroys the (−)ve energy to warm feeling and (+) ve vibes all around.

Then last maha mantra jap [chanting]. It is most powerful in the Vedas. It takes away the fear of death.

Again sit in meditation with shiv mudra and chant the Maha Mrityunjaya Mantra [chant].

OM TRYAMBAKAM YAJAMAHE

SUGANDHIM PUSHTIVARDHANAM

URVARUKAMIVA BANDHANAN

MRITYOR MUKSHIYA MAAMRITAT

End meditation with the sound of the Shankh [shell].
End it with (+) ve energy and slowly open your eyes.
Then rub your palms and put it on your eyes for energy.
Eclipse is a good time for meditation and chanting, when the sun, moon and earth are in the same line, there is a different cosmic energy. The temporary darkening of light, can invite deep, meaningful reflection in our ordinary lives.

Summary

Meditation is very good for the mind, body and soul.

It is your path to happiness, feeling of goodness and wellness.

So experience it and follow it. I enjoy and love to meditate.

Chapter 23

IKIGAII

Having a clearly defined Ikigai brings satisfaction, happiness and meaning to our lives. According to Japanese everyone has Ikiagi-what a French philosopher might call a raison d'être. Some people have found their ikiagi, while others are still looking, though they carry it within them.

This is followed in Okinawa - Japan. It is the island with the most centenarians in the world, their ikiagi is the reason they get up in the morning. It is how people remain active even after they retire.

In fact most never retire. Dan Buettner, a national geographic reporter who knows the country well, having a purpose in life is so important in Japanese culture that the idea of retirement simply doesn't exist there. So do not retire in life

Benefits of Ikigai
They live longer than the rest of the world [100 years].

They suffer fewer chronic illnesses such as cancer and heart disease.

The inflammatory disorders are also less. They enjoy enviable levels of vitality and health that would be unthinkable for people of advanced age elsewhere.

Their blood tests reveal fewer free radicals [which are responsible for cellular aging], as a result of drinking tea and their stomachs are only 80% full.

Both men and women maintain higher levels of sexual hormones much later in life.

Women experience moderate symptoms during menopause. The rate of dementia is well below the global level.

According to scientist the keys of longevity are diet, exercise, finding a purpose in life [an Ikigai], and forming strong social ties - that is having a broad circle of friends and good family relations.

Only staying active will make you want to live a hundred years [Japanese proverb].

BY [RICHELLE E. GOODRICH]
  IT ISN'T ALWAYS A CHANGE OF SCENE
  NEEDED TO MAKE LIFE BETTER,
  SOMETIMES IT SIMPLY REQUIRES
  TO OPEN YOU'RE EYES.

[MITCHELL OBAMA].
  ALWAYS STAY TRUE TO YOURSELF AND

NEVER LET WHAT SOMEBODY ELSE SAYS DISTRACT YOU

Chapter 24

Ozone Therapy

The Oxygen Needed for the Body

This is a very useful adjuvant therapy. Ozone is three molecule of oxygen together. It is extremely good for most of the diseases.
It works wonders in diabetic patients especially in non healing ulcers. It prevents gangrene and saves the part.

I have used it in many patients and they all are happy. The cancer patients are benefited by preventing increase in the tumor size and better health out come.

The Main Action of Ozone is
It opens up the collaterals in spite of your blockages.
It provides more oxygenation to the different parts, as a result the germs are killed.

There is more blood supply also.

It is like cleaning your house.

Thus the heart patients are benefitted. They will not require a bypass. I have seen this myself in many patients.

I have treated the gynecology patients with urinary infection, vaginal infection, infertility. It has amazing action.

Summary
Besides foods, good sleep, happiness, meditation, exercise Ikigai and ozone are important for one.

A man cannot live on water, there are exceptions - right.

You need air, food, family, friends and so on.

So incorporate this into your lifestyle, and be smart and healthy.

Chapter 25

Alcohol and Anti Aging Juices

A] Alcohol

There are seven alcoholic drinks which keeps you healthy and boosts your body. This is partially true drinking alcohol is harmful to the body but only in large and excessive quantity. In fact, despite popular belief moderate drinking (not getting drunk) of good and fine alcohol a few times a week (1 drink per day) with nutrition food is beneficial and good for the general health and longevity.

7 Alcohol Drinks that keep you Secretly Healthy and Going Strong

Beer
The most common alcohol drink beer is loaded with anti-toxins called Phenols. This protects you from heart disease as it is good for circulation. Beer (not more than 2-3 bottles) also lowers risk of high BP and helps in maintaining it.

Red Wine
One of the drinks for ladies and a classy one too, and also having the same beneficial effects of beer. The additional brownie point of red wine is

that it helps in increasing one's life span by generating longevity genes. It is good for cholesterol and reduces bad cholesterol for the body.

Vodka

Vodka when taken in moderate quantity helps in clearing bad breath, as the high alcohol content kills all bad odor. It also helps to reduce stress. It improves the health of the skin and stimulates health growth on the scalp. Vodka indirectly helps toothaches.

Whisky

Whisky when mixed with warm water and used as a gargle does help in relieving throat pain. It helps in preventing dementia, cancer and is healthy for the heart. It increases the level of good cholesterol and terminates blood clots. Whiskey is supposed to be the healthiest drink, amongst all the alcoholic drinks.

Gin

Combination of Gin and Tonic, useful while treating malaria infection as it contains hydroxyl-choloroquine which is also used for treatment in COVID-19

Brandy

Brandy is one alcohol drink which is full of healthy anti-oxidants. It has anti-ageing properties hence very good for the skin. It also reduces the bad cholesterol (LDL) in the body. It helps in sore throat, bladder and ovarian cancer.

Tonic

The combination of gin and tonic is very useful while treating malarial infection as it contains a drug called hydroxychloroquine which is use for the treatment for malaria and now covid-19

Rum

Rum increases life-expectancy/longevity. It is very beneficial drink for the heart. It also works as blood thinner and helps in increasing the level of good cholesterol. This drink guards you against osteoporosis and common cold.

Take Away for Alcoholic Drinks

Drink in Moderation. Never drink too much and take advice of a doctor

It has both bad and good effects.

Daily one peg is better than binging on three four drinks once in a while.

B] Carbonated Drinks

One Must Shout Out a Big No

Carbonated beverages contain dissolved carbon dioxide, which becomes gas when it warms to body temperature in your stomach. So consuming carbonated drink may cause belching, and your stomach stretches from the accumulation of carbon dioxide.

Carbonated drinks increase the risk of diabetes and obesity increases too. It contains a lot of sugars which is harmful, and it increase insulin resistance and stores fat also. Hence blood sugar increases and lots of fat accumulation is there which causes obesity.

Detrimental to Teeth Health
The soda retained in the mouth will actually dissolve the teeth. It even causes the gums to recede causing damage to teeth.

Increased Risk of Rheumatoid Arthritis
The carbon and sugars in the carbonated drin ks leads to this debilating disease and causes joint pains.

Urge to Eat More Foods
It over activates your stomach and invariably you end up eating double than normal. It causes a sense of fullness too.

High in Sugars
Due to its sugar content potent risk of heart disease, diabetes and metabolic syndrome is there.

Take away for Carbonated Drinks
In order to age less you must consume less of the carbonated drinks.

C] Fresh Juices

It is always better to eat fruits than having a glass of juice.

Orange Juice

A glass of orange juice = 4/5 oranges. Eating oranges with its skin gives you a lot of fiber too. It is rich in Vit-C.

Grape Juice

It is rich in Vit-A and Vit-C. Anti ageing effect: It gives a shine to the skin and helps in increasing the collagen and prevents wrinkles.

Carrot Juice

It is rich in carotene and Vit-A.

Eye Health
It improves eyesight.

Anti Ageing Effect
It improvises by increasing collage, thus reducing fine lines.

Skin Benefits
It gives a healthy glow to your skin. It wards off pimples, pigmentation and sun damage.

Beet Root Juice
It is rich in Vit A, Vit-C, Vit K, Folic Acid, Magnesium and iron.

Blood Purifier
The iron in the beet root helps to increase hemoglobin. It carries more oxygen and purifies the blood.

Blood Clotting Effect

The Vit-K helps in the process of clotting of the blood.

Powerful antioxidant
The antioxidant in it prevents the free radicals in the blood. Thus decreases cell damage and anti inflammatory effect on joints.

Tomato Juice

It is rich in Vit C, Vit A and Lycopene along with Vit K, Folate and Potassium.

Hydration Effect of Tomato Juice
The 95% water content of tomatoes helps in hydrating the body and skin. Good for heart health and diabetics

Digestive System and Tomato Juice: Tomatoes are low in carbs and consists of simple sugars and insoluble fibers. The insoluble fibers help in weight reduction and good bowel movement. Thus helps in constipation too.

Oxidative Stress Buster
The lycopene in the tomatoes acts as an oxidative stress buster.

Blood Clotting Effect
The Vit K in tomatoes helps in clotting of the blood and bone health.

Tomatoes are essential for growth of the cells and its function.

Spinach Juice

The benefits of spinach are multiple. It acts as stomach filler. So can be taken as a replacement for meals or can be taken in between the meals. Cucumber, Amla, Alovera juice, lime and orange juice are very beneficial too.

Take Away

Juices are good but better are the fruits.

So you decide fruits or juices.

They hydrate well and have a good effect on people with diarrhea, sunstroke, dizziness, vomiting, and acidity.

D] Beverages - Coffee & Tea

Dr Sanjiv Chopra M.D Physician [Liver Expert] says coffee is most important protector of health. It is an aphrodisiac. Coffee use should be limited one or two cups and do not take it late in the evening.

So people who drank coffee drank had low levels of liver enzymes. They had less fibrosis, a study in the journal of gastroenterology that people who drank two cups of coffee a day had 50% reduction in hospitalization and mortality from chronic liver disorders and 40%reduction in primary liver cancer

Coffee drinkers had low risk of cancers like prostate cancer, colon cancer, skin cancer, endometrial cancer and other diseases like

Parkinsonism disease, cognitive decline, Type 2 Diabetes.

For Type 2 Diabetes one has to drink 6 cups of coffee regularly or decaffeinated coffee then there is 40 to 50% reduction in risk of developing Type 2 Diabetes. Now if somebody has type 2 diabetes and they drink 2 cups of coffee a day regularly, there is a 30% reduction in risk of cardiovascular mortality. Is this not pretty impressive?

The study in the New England Journal of Medicine said men and women who drink coffee have lower total and cause specific mortality.

An article in one of the nutritional journals showed that people who drank coffee have long telomeres. So telomeres were described by Elizabeth Blackburn [an Australian scientist] and she got the Nobel Prize in medicine in physiology in 2009 with two other colleagues. And shortened telomeres are linked with accelerated cellular aging. Who had longer telomeres and by inference they may live longer. A recent study showed that people who drink coffee have longer telomeres.

How much coffee to drink: how many cups to drink? What is the size off cup and whether to drink regular or decaffeinated coffee? One must drink regular coffee which is more better and beneficial then decaffeinated coffee. Don't add sugar or sugar substitutes. I like to drink my coffee black and simple and don't have to worry about sugar and milk.

Sugar substitutes not to be used. It is better to add sugar if you want.

Artificial sugars are turning out to produce worse glucose intolerance because it actually changes the micro biome in the gut and this is one of the hottest topics in medicine. Gut micro biome has been called the second human genome the inner bacterial rainforest.

There are trillions of bacteria in our gastrointestinal tract and in aggregate their weight is 3 pounds. It is a newly discovered organ.

So if you want to have a coca cola, have a Coca-Cola. Maybe have one third, enjoy it, rather than have diet coke which has only 1 calorie but actually has many injuries health effects. Diagnostic detective.com

Summary
Tea too has good benefits and is heart and health friendly.

Always have alcoholic drinks in moderation.

Juices are good. Eating fruits is healthier.

Chapter 26

Conclusion/ End of Story – Don't Eat This Box

MORGAN SPURLOCK SAYS:
SORRY THERE'S NO MAGIC BULLET. YOU GOTTA EAT HEALTHY
AND LIVE HEALTHY TO BE HEALTHY AND LOOK HEALTHY

"

I am very thankful to my mentor Mr. Som Bathla for making my journey as an author possible and easy. Without him I would not have even completed or written this book. Thank you for teaching me self publication and marketing.

NORMAN COUSINS "ANATOMY OF ILLNESS" SAYS:

EACH PATIENT CARRIES HIS OWN DOCTOR INSIDE HIM
THINK GLOBAL BUT EAT LOCAL
DON'T MAKE A HOLE IN YOUR POCKET.
GAME CHANGE PLAN IS EATING IN MODERATION

Water is the elixir of life.

Say goodbye to processed foods.

Try getting most out of your local vendor.

Reduce food wasting.

Take anxiety out of picking what to eat.

Curtail intake of sugar.

Read the labels on food packets. They are deceiving.

Opt for good fats and carbohydrates. Proteins are a must.
Make more use of millets, rather than wheat. Incur less rice daily.

I take millets, rice and chapatti twice/thrice a month.

Eat the plate way, one will never go wrong. Use your kitchen as your medical cabinet.

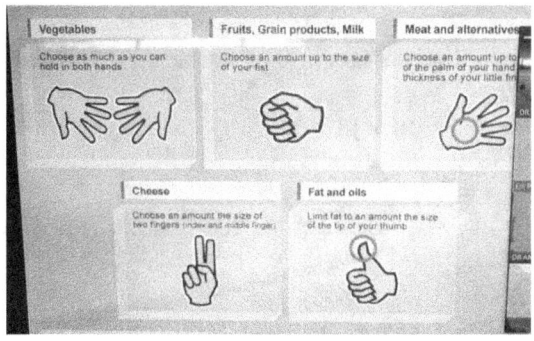

Everyone is processed through the rigmaroles of ageing. Be cautious as to not to fall and hit your head.

Foods are important as they are first basic stepping stone to success.

Low fat milk, spinach and eggs are important for the vegetarian diet.

Don't be hassled about foods, they are all the same. It is a little change here and there. Eat everything that does not make you feel guilty.

Take sensible and balanced, small and frequent meals.

Every meal is important in achieving your fitness goal.

One must create healthy habits and not restrictions.

Bypass junk food for healthy meals.

Make healthy food choices, avoid all fried foods.

Embark on high protein, low carbohydrates, low sugar and high fiber diet.

I am very specific about three things: What I eat, when I eat and how much I eat.

We always eat as we are habituated, meaning what we learn early in our homes and from our parents so make your own recipes to suit you.

My giving you recipes will not serve the purpose, as we are humans and fall back to our original system.

3 C's of Life:
Chances, Choices, Changes. You must take a chance, to make a choice and change your life.

The best investment you can do is your own health.

A healthy outside starts from the inside.

Do not use sugar substitutes.

List of fruits from the sweetest

To the minimally sweet

a] Banana

b] Sapodilla [chiku]

c] Mulberry [shahtoot]

d] Grapes

e] Papaya

f] Custard Apple

g] Water Melon

h] Musk Melon

i] Pear

j] Apple, Green Apple

k] Pineapple

l] Orange

m] Hard Pear

n] Grape Fruit or Wild Berries [bor]

o] Guava

p] Straw Berries

q] Blue Berries]

Notable Quotes

Harriet Beecher Stowe says:
"Never Give Up, For That Is Just
The Place And Time That The Tide Will Turn"

Nelson Mandela says:
"It Always Seem Impossible
Until It's Done"

Chuck Yeager says:
"You Do What You Can For As Long As You Can,
And When You Finally Can't,
You Do The Next Thing.
You Back Up But You Don't Give Up".

Vince Lombardi says:
"Winners never quit,
and quitters never win".

David Schwartz says:
"Believe It Can Be Done.
When You Believe Something Can Be Done,
Really Believe, Your Mind Will Find The Way
To Do It. Believing A Solution Paves The Way
To Solution".

Quick Fixes

Make shot term goals in the beginning, and reward yourself.

Train your mind and make a habit to control over eating.

Try not to eat after dinner and in between meals.

Throw all junk food form the house.

Reduce the intake of sugar.

Take foods with limited salt and the best is Rock Salt.

Cheat diet is okay once in a while.

Do not feel guilty.

Make healthy eating plans your mother taught you.

Foods to Avoid

Do not indulge in different types of diets.

Fat free foods versus sugar free: Both are equally bad.

Biscuits, pastries, cakes, fried foods and diet snacks should say no to them.

Butter and ghee are healthy.

Lifestyle Changes

A] Enjoy more of home cooked foods.

B] Learn to distress yourself.

C] Incur stress management techniques.

D] Good sleep is mandatory.

E] Hydrate yourself well.

F] Become a social animal.

G] Pursue your hobbies.

H] Avoid smoking and drinking alcohol.

I] Make changes to become active and throw the sedentary life style out of the window.

J] Start exercising, go for a walk, move around and sit only when required.

K] Avoid self medication.

L] Farm fresh foods should be your motto.

BE HEALTHY - LOVE THYSELF - CONNECT TO SELF - REMEMBER FOODS ARE THE BASIS TO A HEALTHY DISEASE FREE LIFE

BIBLIOGRAPHY

I have taken the reference from the following books and websites.

For further study you can read about them.

1] www.healthline.com 2www.medicinenet.com 3] www.nhs.uk 4] www.clevaland.com 5] www.webmd.com

6] Clinical Nutrition by Vishwanath Sardesai

7] Dr. Abravanel's Body Type Diet

8] Clinical Dietetics and Nutrition by F.P. Anita and Philip Abraham

9] The Cellulite Solution by Dr. Howard Murad. 10] Think Eat Live smart by dr Anjali Hooda

bone health for osteoporosis and sarcopenia in next edition

.

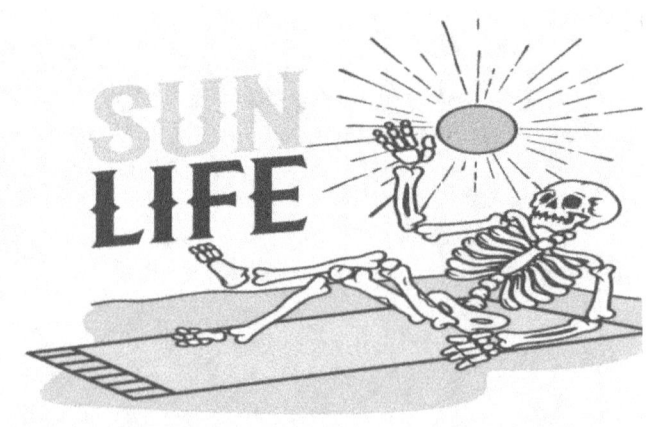

Easy ways with foods, exercise and why it is essential

CONNECTING TO THE AUTHOR

Dr. Maya Modi Shah is a renowned doctor MBBS, DGO, [Gynecologist], FISGE U.K. PGDMLS Pune. I am an Obstetrician and a Gynecologist and a Laparoscopy surgeon. She was the first one to get Laparoscopy in Gujarat and in Vadodara in 1993 at my hospital, Modi Clinic, State of Gujarat, India. She always thought that what she knew and experienced should be shared with many people. The more the people are benefitted the better it would be. It will give the author more joy. This is her first book and she will be coming out with other books too. Bone fixes, Breast health, Women and Menopause. Welcome to the Author's book world, the book full of knowledge, awareness, self care self help and disease free. So enjoy reading this and explore yourself to the best. The author has tried her best to give you the knowledge; some changes may not be there for all the persons.

Ready for help....free for first 100 customers

For any query and discussions, feel free to contact her at:

drmaya53@yahoo.com

"Wishing you a healthy and happy life now and always"

*A JOURNEY, IN WHICH THE PATH IS I,
THE TRAVELER IS ALSO I,
AND SO IS THE DESTINATION.*

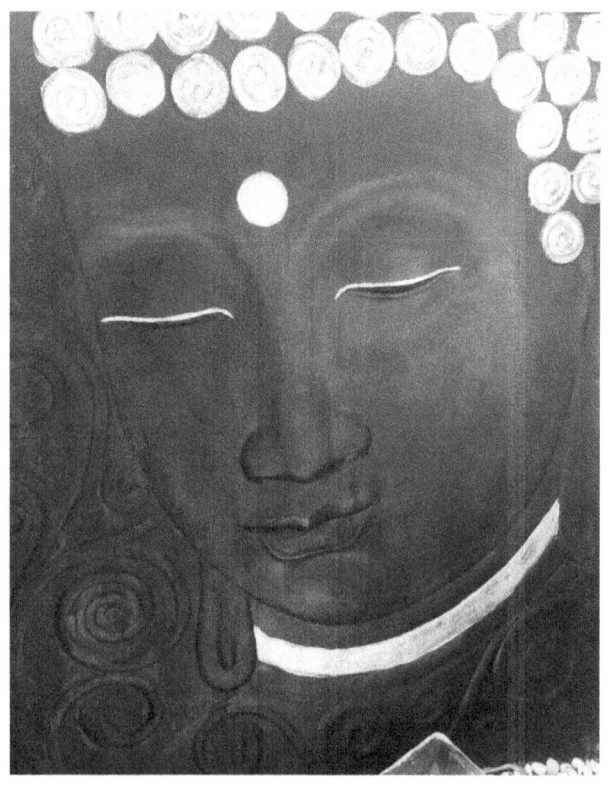

www.ingramcontent.com/pod-product-compliance
Lightning Source LLC
Chambersburg PA
CBHW071350210526
45465CB00001B/47